The Junior Doctor's Guide to Gastroenterology

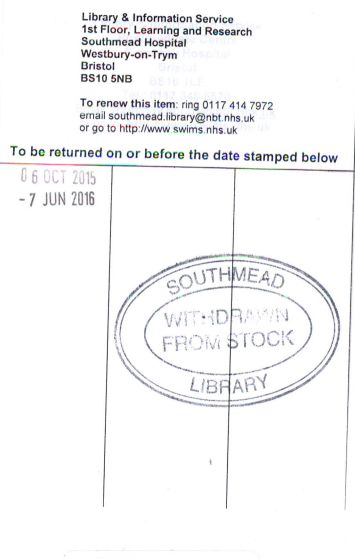

The Junior Doctor's Guide to Gastroenterology

LOUISA BAXTER
MBChB, MRCP, MSc
Academic Clinical Fellow in Public Health
The London School of Hygiene and Tropical Medicine

NEEL SHARMA
BSc (Hons), MBChB, MSc
Core Medical Trainee Year 1
Lewisham Healthcare NHS Trust
and Honorary Clinical Lecturer in Medical Education
Barts and the London School of Medicine and Dentistry

and

IAN MANN
BMedSci (Hons), MBBS, MRCP
Core Medical Trainee Year 2
Royal Brompton Hospital

Foreword by

IAN SANDERSON
Professor of Paediatric Gastroenterology
Director, Digestive Diseases Clinical Academic Unit
Barts and The London NHS Trust

Radcliffe Publishing
London • New York

Radcliffe Publishing Ltd
33–41 Dallington Street
London
EC1V 0BB
United Kingdom

www.radcliffepublishing.com

British Library Cataloguing in Publication Data

A catalogue record for this book is available from the British Library.

ISBN-13: 978 184619 352 1

The paper used for the text pages of this book is FSC® certified. FSC (The Forest Stewardship Council®) is an international network to promote responsible management of the world's forests.

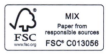

Typeset by Darkriver Design, Auckland, New Zealand
Printed and bound by TJI Digital, Padstow, Cornwall, UK

Contents

Foreword

It is a universal experience in medicine that doctors start on the wards full of knowledge, yet discover that their success rests, to a very large extent, on their practical and organisational skills. In generations past, final year medical students could undertake house officer locums for a few days at a time. This gave some experience; but the governance issues surrounding unqualified medical students working as doctors, now makes this impossible.

There is therefore a gap between what one is taught (the knowledge needed to be a doctor), and what one needs to know to become an efficient junior. This book fills this gap in gastroenterology. The authors have not tried to recapitulate a textbook in gastroenterology, of which many excellent examples are currently available; but they have focused on those practical skills that make for a successful junior doctor. Of course, practical skills are not divorced from background knowledge, and the authors would be the first to point out that each new patient presents an opportunity to learn. Out-of-work study on the clinical conditions in each patient is richly rewarding for junior doctors, and for the care of future patients.

Because this is a practical handbook, the authors have not included sections on how to write a history, take daily notes and how to organise a succinct discharge summary. But this is not to underestimate the importance of these aspects of the job. These pieces of writing remain in the notes for many years and are widely read.

I know the reader will find this book very helpful. The authors have distilled their experiences in working as young doctors into a concise format. I certainly wish I had had such an aid when I was a gastroenterology house physician.

Professor Ian Sanderson
Director, Digestive Diseases Clinical Academic Unit
Barts and The London NHS Trust
July 2011

Preface

Becoming a first year doctor is a stressful time as you make the transition from the relatively sheltered life of a medical student. You are suddenly a member of a medical team with responsibilities that far outstrip those of the normal young professional. This can be a difficult time for even the most competent junior doctors. To add to the stress and pressure, junior doctors are expected to rotate around different medical specialties every 4 to 6 months, and to possess a well-grounded understanding from day one on the job. They often feel as if they are outside their comfort zone, and are commonly too embarrassed to ask for help or advice.

The majority of the books that are currently available are packed full of information, but much of this is not aimed at junior doctors working on the front line. These books often list countless investigations and areas of management for specific medical conditions. However, they lack an explanation of what results you should expect to obtain from these investigations and the interpretation in the clinical context. We have written this book for junior doctors in the hope that it will act as a 'user's guide' for day-to-day clinical gastroenterology while out on the wards. It is designed to provide a logical stepwise guide through the more common problems encountered in gastroenterology, and to support you in your clinical practice and decision making.

The book is primarily aimed at FY1 and FY2 doctors, to act as a means of quick reference on the ward. We hope that it will provide you with some user-friendly support which you can use in your daily clinical practice, and that it will make life slightly more comfortable for both you and your patients. Good luck!

Ian Mann
Louisa Baxter
Neel Sharma
July 2011

About the authors

Dr Louisa Baxter graduated from Manchester University in 2003. She completed her House Officer rotation at Central Manchester University Hospital, and subsequently moved to St Bartholomew's and the Royal London Hospitals as a Senior House Officer.

She went on to gain her MRCP in 2005, and worked as a Gastroenterology Specialist Registrar at King's College Hospital in the liver transplant unit. At the same time she completed an MSc in management with a special interest in health policy at the London School of Economics. More recently she spent a year in the USA as a Commonwealth Fund Harkness Fellow. She is currently furthering her interest in public health as an Academic Clinical Fellow at the London School of Hygiene and Tropical Medicine.

Dr Neel Sharma graduated from Manchester University School of Medicine in 2007. He completed his foundation training in the North East Thames region, and subsequently completed a Master's degree in Gastroenterology at St Bartholomew's and the Royal London School of Medicine and Dentistry. He is currently undertaking core medical training at Lewisham Healthcare NHS Trust and has been appointed as Honorary Clinical Lecturer in Medical Education.

Dr Ian Mann graduated from St Bartholomew's and the Royal London School of Medicine and Dentistry in 2007, with distinctions in Clinical Practice and Clinical Science. He also obtained a first-class Biomedical Sciences degree with honours in Molecular Therapeutics during his intercalated year at medical school. He then went on to gain his MRCP in November 2010 while working on the intensive-care unit at the Royal Brompton Hospital.

He is currently working in cardiology at the Royal Brompton Hospital in his second year of the Core Medical Training Programme, and is about to continue his training in London as a Specialist Registrar in Cardiology. Dr Mann has a particular interest in electrophysiology, as well as in general cardiology. He is also interested in medical education, and dedicates a large amount of his time to the ward-based teaching of medical students and nursing staff.

List of abbreviations

ABC	Airway, breathing, circulation
ABG	Arterial blood gas
AFB	Acid-fast bacilli
AIDS	Acquired immunodeficiency syndrome
AIH	Autoimmune hepatitis
ALF	Acute liver failure
ALP	Alkaline phosphatase
ALT	Alanine transaminase
AMA	Anti-mitochondrial antibodies
ANA	Anti-nuclear antibodies
ANCA	Anti-neutrophil cytoplasmic antibodies
Anti-SMA	Anti-smooth muscle antibodies
AP	Anterior-posterior
APTT	Activated partial thromboplastin time
ASA	Aminosalicylic acid
ASMA	Anti-smooth muscle antibodies
AST	Aspartate transaminase
AXR	Abdominal X-ray
BBV	Blood-borne virus
BD	Bis in die (twice a day)
BNF	*British National Formulary*
BP	Blood pressure
BSG	British Society of Gastroenterology
cAMP	Cyclic adenosine monophosphate
CBD	Common bile duct
CD	Crohn's disease
CDAI	Crohn's Disease Activity Index
CEA	Carcinoembryonic antigen
CFTR	Cystic fibrosis transmembrane receptor
CMV	Cytomegalovirus
COPD	Chronic obstructive pulmonary disease
CRP	C-reactive protein
CT	Computed tomography
CXR	Chest X-ray

DIC	Disseminated intravascular coagulation
DRE	Digital rectal examination
DSA	Digital subtraction angiography
DVT	Deep vein thrombosis
EBV	Epstein–Barr virus
ECG	Electrocardiogram
ERCP	Endoscopic retrograde cholangiopancreatography
ESR	Erythrocyte sedimentation rate
ET	Endo-tracheal
EUS	Endoscopic ultrasound
FAP	Familial adenomatous polyposis
FBC	Full blood count
FFP	Fresh frozen plasma
GCS	Glasgow Coma Scale
GGT	Gamma-glutamyl transpeptidase
GI	Gastrointestinal
GORD	Gastro-oesophageal reflux disease
GP	General practitioner
HAS	Human albumin solution
HAV	Hepatitis A virus
Hb	Haemoglobin
HCV	Hepatitis C virus
HDU	High dependency unit
HEV	Hepatitis E virus
HIV	Human immunodeficiency virus
HLA	Human leukocyte antigen
HNPCC	Hereditary non-polyposis colorectal cancer
HRS	Hepatorenal syndrome
IBD	Inflammatory bowel disease
IBS	Irritable bowel syndrome
ICP	Intracranial pressure
INR	International normalised ratio
ITU	Intensive treatment unit
IUD	Intrauterine device
IV	Intravenous
IVC	Inferior vena cava
IVP	Intravenous pyelogram
IVU	Intravenous urogram
LDH	Lactate dehydrogenase
LFTs	Liver function tests
LLQ	Left lower quadrant
LMP	Last menstrual period

LUQ	Left upper quadrant
MC&S	Microscopy, culture and sensitivity
MDT	Multidisciplinary team
MELD	Model for End-Stage Liver Disease
MRCP	Magnetic resonance cholangiopancreatography
MRI	Magnetic resonance imaging
MSU	Midstream urine
NAC	N-acetyl cysteine
NAFLD	Non-alcoholic fatty liver disease
NBM	Nil by mouth
NG	Nasogastric
NICE	National Institute for Health and Clinical Excellence
NSAIDs	Non-steroidal anti-inflammatory drugs
O&G	Obstetrics and gynaecology
OGD	Oesophagogastroduodenoscopy
pANCA	Perinuclear anti-neutrophil cytoplasmic antibodies
PBC	Primary biliary cirrhosis
PCR	Polymerase chain reaction
PCV	Polcythaemia rubra vera
PET	Positron emission tomography
PID	Pelvic inflammatory disease
PLT	Platelet
PO	Per os (by mouth)
PPI	Proton pump inhibitor
PR	Per rectum
PT	Prothrombin time
PTH	Parathyroid hormone
PUD	Peptic ulcer disease
QDS	Quater die sumendus (four times a day)
RLQ	Right lower quadrant
RUQ	Right upper quadrant
SAAG	Serum-ascites albumin gradient
SBP	Systolic blood pressure; spontaneous bacterial peritonitis
SRH	Stigmata of recent haemorrhage
TIBC	Total iron-binding capacity
TLOSRs	Transient lower oesophageal sphincter relaxations
TNM	Tumour, Node, Metastasis
TPMT	Thiopurine methyltransferase
TSH	Thyroid-stimulating hormone
UC	Ulcerative colitis
U&E	Urea and electrolytes
UGIB	Upper gastrointestinal bleeding

US	Ultrasound
USS	Ultrasound scan
UTI	Urinary tract infection
VIP	Vasoactive intestinal peptide
WCC	White cell count
WHO	World Health Organization

Targeted gastroenterology examination

The gastrointestinal system extends from the lips to the anus, and includes the pancreas and hepatobiliary system. A complete GI examination includes a digital rectal examination (DRE) and examination of hernial orifices; it may also include pelvic examination. Vomitus, stool and urine samples should be inspected. The patient's observation chart, as well as radiological studies and laboratory investigations, must also be considered part of the routine examination.

Introduction

It is vital to ensure patient comfort and privacy during the clinical examination. The examination room should be warm, well lit, and have adequate supplies of examination gloves, lubricant and tissues.

There is no consensus on the use of chaperones during the physical examination. We suggest that a chaperone of the same sex as the patient should always be utilised if the patient accepts this. This will usually be a member of the nursing staff or a fellow clinician. Family members should be asked to leave the examination room unless the patient requests otherwise.

Obtain verbal consent to examine the patient, and explain what the examination entails. A translator should be used for a patient whose first language is not that of the examiner if there are any concerns about understanding.

It is traditional to examine the patient from the right-hand side. Ask the patient to adopt the supine position if this is comfortable. The bed should be flat and positioned at the level of the examiner's hip. To ensure that the abdominal wall is fully relaxed, remove the pillows behind the patient's head. If this is uncomfortable, a thin pillow may be left in place.

Patients should undress themselves without assistance from the doctor unless for any reason they are unable to do so. It is suggested that the patient should remain draped during the general examination, and should then be exposed from nipples to knees for the targeted examination.

Inspection

- Throughout the examination it is vital to observe the patient's face for signs of discomfort.
- The patient and the environment around them should be inspected from the end of the bed. Look carefully for signs of muscle wasting or weight loss, such as redundant skin folds. Is there evidence of jaundice, poor mobility or use of living aids?
- Approach the patient more closely. Do they appear to be in pain or distress? Are they comfortable lying flat? Is there evidence of neglect, or of alcohol misuse?
- A formal examination should begin with the patient's hands. Look for signs of tar staining from cigarette smoking, leukonychia from chronic illness indicating hypoalbuminaemia, and koilonychia associated with iron deficiency. Assess the warmth of the hands and the rate and rhythm of the pulse. Also assess the capillary refill time, and look for signs of haemodynamic instability. Assess for a liver flap.
- Inspect the patient's face for indications of their state of hydration and nutrition. Look for evidence of jaundice. Angular stomatitis may be evidence of vitamin deficiencies.
- The torso should be inspected for scars, signs of visible peristalsis, redundant skin folds, abdominal masses and evidence of chronic liver disease (e.g. loss of normal hair distribution, gynaecomastia, etc.).

Palpation

- Division of the abdomen into either four quadrants or nine regions is recommended. Before palpation ask the patient if they are experiencing any pain, and if so where.
- Examine each quadrant in turn, starting with light palpation. Look for signs of tenderness and assess for guarding. Use deeper palpation to identify abdominal masses or areas of deep tenderness.
- Palpate the liver, starting in the right iliac fossa. Time palpation with the patient's respiratory cycle.
- Palpate the spleen, again starting in the right iliac fossa. A normal healthy spleen should not be palpable.
- Ballot the kidneys. An enlarged kidney should be palpable by the anterior hand.

- Rebound tenderness is used to test for evidence of peritoneal irritation, and may be uncomfortable for the patient. It is advisable to warn them before proceeding. Press deeply on the abdomen with your hand, hold for a moment and then quickly release. Rebound tenderness is indicated by increased pain on release of pressure rather than on applying it.
- Tenderness in the renal angle may indicate inflammation of the kidneys (e.g. pyelonephritis). Again assessment of this may be uncomfortable, so warn the patient. Ask them to sit up, and then using your hand tap firmly in both costophrenic angles.

Percussion

- **Liver.** Percuss down from the chest in the anterior right mid-clavicular line until you detect the top border of liver dullness. Percussion should be repeated from the right iliac fossa upward until the lower border of liver dullness is detected. The distance between these two points should be measured. The normal distance in an adult is in the range 6–12 cm.
- **Spleen.** Percuss the lowest costal space in the left anterior axillary line. This area is normally tympanitic. Ask the patient to take a deep breath and percuss this area again. Dullness in this area is a sign of splenic enlargement. Again, you should also percuss the spleen from the right iliac fossa towards the left upper quadrant.
- **Shifting dullness.** This will assess for the presence of peritoneal fluid (ascites). Percuss the patient's abdomen to outline areas of dullness and tympany. Percuss across the abdomen, noting the point of transition from tympany to dullness. Then roll the patient on their side away from the examiner, and repeat percussion from the umbilicus to the flank area. When ascites is present, the area of dullness will shift to the dependent site. The area of tympany will shift towards the top.

Auscultation

Use the diaphragm of the stethoscope on the anterior abdominal wall. Auscultate for bowel sounds and bruits over the renal arteries, iliac arteries and aorta.

The digital rectal examination

- Inspect the perianal area for tags, fissures, excoriations, etc.
- Lubricate your gloved index finger and warn the patient before inserting the finger.

- Gently press on the sphincter's edge and wait for it to relax, and then insert your finger into the anal canal. Assess sphincter tone by asking the patient to squeeze their anal muscles around your finger.
- Examine the posterior and lateral walls of the rectum by gently rotating the finger through 180 degrees.
- Palpate the entire circumference of the rectum. You should turn away from the patient and hyper-pronate your wrist to do this effectively. Sweep your finger across the anterior and anterolateral walls of the rectum and note the texture of the rectal mucosa, which should be smooth and non-tender.
- Inspect the gloved finger for stool colour, melaena, blood, mucus and pus.

Successful ward rounds in gastroenterology

Preparation and organisation are the cornerstones to achieving a successful ward round. However, more than this is required in order to provide the best possible care for the patient. Your consultant may well be pleased if you are able to competently organise a ward round, but will be less than impressed if you send a patient for an ERCP without stopping their warfarin.

Time management

Time management is an important aspect of any doctor's working life, and a skill that should be learned early on in your career. It encompasses the ability to organise, plan, prioritise and budget time so as to improve the effectiveness of work and increase productivity. This is especially important in the context of a ward round, as it may have direct ramifications for patient care.

There are several key areas on which you need to focus. It is important to bear these points in mind when doing any ward round, whether it is a consultant or registrar round, or your own ward round.

Up-to-date patient list

It is easy to adopt a lackadaisical approach to producing a patient list, but this will only make your own life more difficult. The following important information should be included on your patient list:

- patient details (name, date of birth and hospital number)
- ward number
- bed number
- admission complaint and past medical history
- current problems and management
- jobs, including investigations to book, results to chase, etc.

Who to review first

It is tempting to review all of the easy patients first, and leave the more complex ones to concentrate on later. However, you should always see the sickest patients first. This will mean that any potential problems will be recognised earlier in the day, leaving more time in which to contact the relevant people in an attempt to rectify the situation. It is best to categorise patients into one of the three groups listed below, and see them in the following order:

1   sickest patients
2   new patients – as you have never met the patients in this group, you will not know anything about their general condition. They are also likely to require investigative and management plans, which can be complex and time consuming to arrange
3   stable patients – this patient group should be further subdivided as follows:
    * stable but requiring further treatment
    * medically fit for discharge.

Investigations and procedures

Once the decision has been made to request an investigation or procedure, then depending on what is being requested it may take some time to organise. Bearing this in mind, the sooner it is requested, the more quickly it is likely to happen. For example, if it is decided at 10am on a ward round that a patient requires a CT scan, fill in the form at the time and hand it in as soon as possible. If you finish the ward round, go off for lunch and finally hand in the request at 3 pm, it is highly unlikely that the scan will take place that day. At best it will be done the following day. You may find that the scan could have been done on the same day if the request had been handed in earlier. The end result will involve prolonging patient care and lengthening their hospital stay.

When going to departments to request investigations and procedures, ask yourself whether they are urgent or non-urgent. If they are urgent, always go and discuss them with the relevant person who will actually be performing the investigation or procedure. Not only is this a matter of common courtesy, but also you may be able to negotiate for your investigation or procedure to be performed sooner. Other important factors to bear in mind when making your request include the following:

* Understand what you are requesting.
* Understand what you are trying to prove or disprove. If you are not sure, ask your seniors before making the request. Saying 'My consultant wanted me to ask for this scan' never goes down particularly well!
* Is what you are requesting appropriate, or even possible? If you are requesting a non-urgent gastroscopy for a patient who has had a

troponin-positive cardiac event 3 days previously, your request will be refused. This is because a non-urgent gastroscopy must be performed at least 6 weeks after a troponin-positive cardiac event.
- Has the patient had the appropriate preparation?

Discharge summaries

There is no reason why a discharge summary cannot be started upon admission of the patient. Throughout their admission it can be updated, and this will avoid the last-minute panic of rushing to prepare a poor-quality discharge summary 10 minutes before transport services are due to collect the patient to take them home. Discharge summaries are extremely important, as they provide the GP with vital information about what has happened during the admission. Furthermore, if any future admissions to the hospital are required, they provide a good background history.

Working relationships

Medicine is fully established as a multi-disciplinary environment where many different health professionals work together to provide a high quality of care for the patient. In the context of gastroenterology, the multi-disciplinary team (MDT) is extensive and includes the following:
- doctors (consultant, registrar, junior doctors)
- upper and lower GI surgeons, hepatobiliary surgeons
- nursing staff
- specialist nurses (IBD nurse, stoma nurse, nutrition nurse specialist, Macmillan nurse, etc.)
- pharmacists
- radiologists
- physiotherapists
- social workers
- occupational therapists
- bed managers
- secretaries.

It is important to recognise each individual's role and contribution to the team, and the importance that this has for providing high-quality patient care. When you start out as a newly qualified or junior doctor, it is important to recognise that some senior nursing staff will have over 20 years of experience. As a result, their knowledge will prove invaluable. Don't turn up on day one and upset or annoy them, as this will only make your own life more difficult, as well as compromising patient care.

When you start, you should introduce yourself to the various members of the MDT and make a point of remembering their names. This will make you more approachable, and will also prove beneficial when, for example, you are trying to organise an OGD. People will be more willing to stay on for a few minutes at the end of the day to squeeze your patient on to their list if you are polite and have built up a good rapport with them. A great deal of this may seem obvious, but it is surprising how often it is forgotten or overlooked.

Presenting on ward rounds

Presenting a patient on a ward round involves more than just reading from the notes. More often than not, consultant ward rounds take place on a pre-organised day and at a pre-arranged time, so there should be no excuse for being unprepared.

Preparing for the ward round

You should start to prepare for the ward round about an hour before it is due to begin. This will allow you plenty of time to make sure that you have everything ready. A good-quality ward round is one in which you, as the junior, lead your team round the patients, presenting them as you go. We shall break down the process of preparation into categories, each of which is described below.

Patient list

Make sure that you have an up-to-date patient list (as discussed previously), and print off enough copies for everyone who will be on the ward round. Remember to prioritise the order in which the patients are seen!

Bloods folder

- A flow-sheet of blood results from admission is essential. Make sure that this is up to date with the latest results. It is often best to do this before you leave work the previous day, as you must always see blood results on the same day that they are requested. If the results are not going to be back by the time you finish work, hand them over to the on-call doctor to check, together with a plan.
- If a patient is anaemic, look back to see whether this is a new or old finding, and whether it has been appropriately investigated.

Results

Search on the computers and through the old notes for any recent and old investigations and procedures that the patient has had which are relevant to their current admission. Ensure that you read through the results so that you can present them on the ward round.

Old letters

Old clinic letters provide a vast amount of information about care that the patient has previously received. They also provide information about other consultants to whom the patient is known, and the management that they are receiving from them. In addition, old letters can be important in the context of further management, investigations and the ceiling of care.

New patients

Read through the notes of the new patients to find out the reason for admission, what the management plan is, and what has been done to date. It may also be worth 'eyeballing' the patients from the end of the bed to get a crude idea of their general condition.

Old notes

Old notes provide extremely useful information. However, it can often be difficult to get hold of them. As soon as a patient is admitted, it is worth speaking to the ward clerk to ask them to request the old notes, in order to minimise any delays in obtaining them.

Charts

Just before the ward round is due to start, go round all of your patients and open the observation charts and drug charts at the end of the bed so that they are ready for the consultant to review. If you are running about trying to track down where the charts have gone, not only does this waste time but also it looks unprofessional.

Talking to families and patients

This aspect of medicine is often completely overlooked, but is arguably one of the most important areas. Many of us are extremely busy, but this should not prevent us from setting aside time to explain what is happening to both the patient and their family.

Before you discuss any information with a patient you must ascertain what, if anything, they want to know. On occasion you will meet patients who do not wish to know about any aspect of their illness. In all cases you must always gain the patient's consent before any discussion with their family.

Daily updates

A brief update on a daily basis during the ward round is a good way to explain the current plan for the patient, and also to gauge how the patient feels about this. Updating and explaining the results of any investigations and discussing the plan for any further investigations will go a long way towards alleviating the anxiety of both the patient and their family.

After your daily update, ask the patient and their family whether they have any questions. This will ensure that everything has been covered. These brief updates are extremely reassuring for patients, and will also help to prevent lengthy discussions with dissatisfied relatives.

Formal discussions

On occasion it is not appropriate to give the patient or their family a brief update on the ward. The classic example is, of course, breaking bad news. In this instance it is important to set time aside. A specific time should be arranged that is convenient for both parties. It is essential that you find a more private area than the open ward. Switch off your bleep, or hand it to a colleague. Take time to discuss any information, and invite questions. After any discussion, it may be appropriate to ask the patient and their family if they would like to remain in the same room for a short time after you have left.

Documentation

This is usually very poorly done in practice. Documentation of any discussions will be extremely useful if there is any dispute, and for ensuring that on-call teams are aware of the current situation and what the patient knows.

Daily updates should be included in the ward-round notes, and need only be brief. Any formal discussions should be clearly documented with the following information:

- date and time of discussion
- the names of all individuals present at the discussion. Document the names of family members, e.g. 'Jane Smith', rather than just 'sister'. The patient may have four sisters, one of whom is estranged!
- the information given and general level of explanation
- any questions or concerns raised by the patient or their family.

3

Introduction to specialist investigations and procedures

Inserting a nasogastric tube

A nasogastric (NG) tube is a narrow-bore tube that is passed into the stomach through the nasal cavity. It may be used to aspirate the stomach contents (e.g. to decompress the stomach if bowel obstruction is suspected) and to provide nutritional support. It may also be used to introduce certain medications. NG tubes that are inserted to feed patients are thinner than the wide-bore Ryles tubes that are used for drainage.

NG tube placement is contraindicated in patients with nasal injuries and base-of-skull fractures, as the tube may be misplaced in these patients and cause damage to local structures. All NG tubes may cause nasal irritation and oesophageal erosions.

Prepare the patient
- Explain the procedure to the patient and obtain their consent.
- It is suggested that an assistant should be present (a nurse or another doctor).
- Suggest a signal for the patient to use to stop the procedure (e.g. 'Raise your right hand if it gets too uncomfortable').
- Have suction set up on hand to remove secretions if necessary.
- Sit the patient in a semi-upright position with their head supported with pillows.
- Make sure that a vomit bowl is available in case the procedure triggers emesis.

Equipment
- Protective clothing (sterile gloves, apron, protective eye mask).
- Suction.
- Oxygen mask.
- Lubricant.
- Cup of water and straw.
- Vomit bowl.
- NG tube, and tape to secure it.
- Syringe, litmus paper and indicator (most hospitals will have pre-packed kits containing these items).

Procedure
- Take universal precautions (apron, mask, gloves).
- Examine both nostrils for deformity or obstructions, in order to determine the best side for insertion.
- Measure the NG tubing from the bridge of the nose to the earlobe, and then to the point halfway between the lower end of the sternum and the navel.
- Mark the measured length with a marker, or make a note of the measurement.
- Lubricate 2–5 cm of tube (e.g. with 2% Xylocaine).
- Pass the tube via either nostril, past the pharynx, into the oesophagus and then into the stomach. If the patient swallows this may aid the passage of the tube. Providing the patient with a glass of water and a straw through which to sip this may be useful if aspiration is not a significant concern.
- If the tube will not pass any further, ensure that it is not coiled in the back of the mouth, and then try rotating it slowly. If this fails, reattempt the procedure using the other nostril. Stop and pull back the tube if the patient becomes distressed, starts to cough or gasp, or withdraws consent.
- Pass the tube until the reference mark is reached.
- Confirm the tube position at this point and secure it.
- Remove the inner guide wire.

Checking tube position
- The tube position must be confirmed prior to use.
- The gold standard test is pH testing of gastric aspirate. Aspirate a small amount (1–2 ml) of fluid from the tube and place this on litmus paper. Correct placement is indicated by a pH of < 4, but it may be in the range pH 4–6 if the patient is receiving gastric acid suppressants.
- X-rays will only confirm the position of the tube at the time of

the X-ray, so are not an ideal means of confirming placement. It is important to note that the tube may shift with patient movement. Leave the guide wire in if you are sending the patient for X-ray confirmation to aid visibility.

- The traditional test that involves introducing a small quantity of air into the stomach and then checking for a bubbling sound over the epigastrium is not recommended as it is unreliable and can give false reassurance.

Abdominal paracentesis

This is performed as a diagnostic procedure to evaluate the aetiology of ascites, or as a treatment for tense ascites (massive fluid accumulation which may be interfering with breathing). Paracentesis may be performed 'blind' or under direct visualisation by ultrasound in the radiology department.

Abdominal paracentesis is contraindicated in patients with coagulopathy or thrombocytopenia, in pregnant women, and in patients with infection of the abdominal wall or intestinal obstruction. It requires a high level of patient cooperation, so may not be suitable for all individuals. Patients who have had multiple abdominal surgeries and/or multiple previous abdominal paracenteses may benefit from a US-guided procedure, as scarring may make blind insertion technically difficult.

Prepare the patient

- Check the FBC, clotting and platelet count prior to the procedure. Ascites is a sign of chronic liver disease, so these parameters may be deranged. Guidelines suggest that it is safe to perform paracentesis if the platelet count is > 70×10^9/l and the INR is < 1.5. If these values are deranged they may need to be corrected prior to the procedure with platelets and fresh frozen plasma (FFP). If these products are required, discuss this with your senior and the haematology laboratory. Both of these products have a short half-life, so the paracentesis must take place within 1 hour of both products being received.
- Explain the risks, benefits and details of the procedure to the patient prior to obtaining their consent. Complications include the introduction of infection, needle injury to intra-abdominal structures, bleeding and abdominal wall haematoma. Large-volume paracentesis may cause haemodynamic instability.
- Position the patient in the bed with their head elevated to an angle of 45–90 degrees. This allows fluid to accumulate in the lower abdomen.
- It is suggested that you have an assistant available.

Equipment
- Protective clothing (sterile gloves, apron, eye mask).
- Drapes.
- Wound care pack.
- Iodine scrub.
- Sterile gauze.
- Local anaesthetic (1% lidocaine) and needles.
- Syringes: 2 × 10 ml, 2 × 50 ml.
- Paracentesis needles:
  - 16-, 18- and 20-gauge
  - spinal needle (18- and 20-gauge) for obese patients.
- Sterile specimen tubes.
- Blood culture bottles.
- Biochemistry bottle for glucose.
- Bonanno catheter (or ascitic drain) and catheter bag and connections (for therapeutic procedures).
- Tape and sterile scissors.

Procedure for diagnostic paracentesis
- This procedure requires an aseptic technique.
- Identify the point of aspiration. This is usually in the midline, avoiding prominent veins and midway between the umbilicus and the pubis (to avoid the inferior epigastric artery). If scars from previous surgery are present, choose the right or left lower quadrant lateral to the rectus muscles.
- Sterilise the site with iodine solution, using a circular technique. Site sterile drapes.
- Draw up 5 ml of lidocaine with a green needle. Exchange the needle for a smaller-gauge needle (blue or orange), and inject lidocaine down to and including the peritoneum.
- Insert an 18- to 20-gauge needle on a 10-ml syringe slowly into the abdominal cavity at a slightly oblique angle to the skin after pulling the skin down slightly (the so-called 'Z-track technique', which may reduce the risk of ascites leaks), and aspirate intermittently.
- Gently aspirate 10 ml of fluid, and then attach the 50-ml syringe and aspirate further quantities of fluid as needed for predetermined analysis (usually 20–200 ml).
- If no fluid returns after several attempts, ultrasound-directed aspiration should be used.
- Remove the needle and place an adhesive dressing over the site.

Procedure for therapeutic paracentesis

- Prepare the patient as for a diagnostic procedure.
- In patients for whom a large-volume paracentesis is planned, 100 ml of 20% human albumin solution (HAS) are given intravenously for every 2 litres of ascitic fluid removed, to balance fluid shifts. If HAS is required, this must be discussed with the pharmacists and prescribed on the fluid chart. It is wise not to begin paracentesis until the HAS has been prepared, in order to prevent any delay in its administration.
- Prepare the Bonanno catheter. Remove the plastic tip at the end.
- Once the needle is in place and you have confirmed a flow of ascitic fluid, remove the needle and introduce the Bonanno catheter tip at the same point using the Seldinger technique, pulling back the metal guide wire as the plastic tubing remains in the abdominal cavity. Ascitic fluid should be visible at the end of the port. If it is not, reattach the syringe and aspirate.
- Attach one end of the tubing to the end of the port and the other end of the tubing to the collection bag. To keep the drain in place, cut a slit in the gauze and tape this around the site. The patient must be advised to mobilise with caution and to ensure that the collection bag remains below the level of the drain site, in order to optimise drainage.
- Drains should not be left in place for more than 6 hours. Remove the gauze and gently withdraw the Bonanno catheter. Apply pressure and then apply a dressing to the site.
- Monitor the patient's observations closely during a large-volume drain, to avoid hypotension.

Ascitic fluid analysis

Routine tests for ascitic fluid analysis include the following:

1 **Total protein and albumin.** This is traditionally used to decide whether ascites is an exudate (> 25 g/l) or a transudate (< 25 g/l). The serum-ascites albumin gradient (SAAG) is a better measure (see below).
2 **Microscopy.** This is used to screen for spontaneous bacterial peritonitis (SBP), which occurs in approximately 15% of patients with cirrhosis and ascites who are admitted to hospital. An ascitic neutrophil count of > 250 cells/mm^3 is diagnostic of SBP.
3 **Microscopy.** Red blood cell count should be measured, as bloody ascites may indicate a traumatic tap. In about one-third of cirrhotic patients with bloody ascites there is an underlying hepatocellular carcinoma.
4 **Gram and acid-fast bacillus stain.**
5 **Amylase.** Levels will be raised in pancreatic ascites.
6 **Culture (bacterial, acid-fast bacilli, fungal and viral).** The best method is to inoculate blood culture bottles with ascitic fluid at the bedside. This

will identify an organism in approximately 70% of cases of SBP, whereas sending ascitic fluid in a sterile container to the laboratory will only identify an organism in about 40% of cases.

7   **Cytology.** Sending a large volume of ascites (e.g. 200–300 ml) increases the accuracy of cytological examination in the diagnosis of malignant ascites.

The serum-ascites albumin gradient (SAAG)

A high gradient (> 1.1 g/dl) indicates with 97% accuracy that the ascites is due to portal hypertension.

Causes of high SAAG ascites (> 1.1 g/dl) include the following:

- > 2.5: heart failure
- < 2.5: cirrhosis of the liver, Budd–Chiari syndrome.

A low gradient (< 1.1 g/dl) indicates ascites that is not associated with increased portal pressure. Causes of this include nephrotic syndrome, tuberculosis and malignancy.

Endoscopy

Upper GI endoscopy (oesophagogastroduodenoscopy/gastroscopy)

This is an examination of the inside of the oesophagus, stomach and first part of the duodenum using a thin fibre-optic endoscope that is passed through the mouth. It is performed either under light sedation or with topical anaesthetics (throat spray). Diagnostic gastroscopy is indicated to investigate dyspepsia, abdominal pain, dysphagia, anaemia, weight loss, persistent vomiting and haematemesis, and to take biopsies of the upper GI mucosa. Therapeutic endoscopy is used to treat bleeding from the upper GI tract and difficulties with swallowing.

Gastroscopy is performed by gastroenterologists or upper GI surgeons, and many non-urgent cases are undertaken in an outpatient or day-case setting. Junior doctors (house officers and senior house officers) will not be required to perform endoscopy or consent patients for the procedure. However, they will be expected to know about the preparation of patients for endoscopy, and their aftercare.

Gastroscopy is contraindicated in patients who have recently had an acute myocardial infarction (within the last 6 weeks), who are hypoxic with respiratory distress, who are hypotensive and shocked, and in those with massive upper GI bleeding with hypotension, where emergency surgery is more appropriate. Gastroscopy is also contraindicated in cases of acute peritonitis, perforation of an abdominal viscus, and severe coagulopathy.

The complications of gastroscopy include damage to the GI tract from the endoscope, leading to perforation and bleeding and the introduction of infection. In addition, respiratory depression caused by the use of sedation may occur. The most common side-effect is a transient sore throat. Complications may be obvious immediately following the procedure, or may be delayed. Complication rates are higher in the elderly and during therapeutic procedures.

Prepare the patient

- Check the FBC, clotting and platelet count prior to the procedure. Guidelines suggest that it is safe to perform gastroscopy and biopsy if the platelet count is $> 70 \times 10^9/l$ and the INR is < 1.5.
- The patient should be nil by mouth from midnight the night before the procedure. This is to reduce the risk of vomiting and enable a better examination of the GI tract. Morning medications should be omitted, and patients at particular risk from dehydration, such as the elderly, should be commenced on maintenance IV fluids (e.g. 1 litre of 0.9% sodium chloride over 8–10 hours).
- The nurse in charge of the endoscopy department should be informed about any diabetic patients before the procedure, so that these patients can be placed first on the list. Patients who are taking oral hypoglycaemic agents should omit their morning dose.
- Most antiplatelet and anticoagulant drugs should be stopped before the procedure. This must be discussed with your consultant and the endoscopy department when listing the patient, as failure to comply with endoscopy guidelines may result in a test being cancelled. Particular caution is needed when stopping clopidogrel treatment in patients with coronary artery stents. This must be discussed with your seniors.
- Patients with metallic cardiac valve replacements will pose significant challenges with regard to anticoagulation, and must be discussed with your seniors.

Aftercare

1 Following endoscopy, patients who have been sedated will be transferred to a recovery area in the department for observation. Patients who have received anaesthetic throat spray are usually returned to the ward sooner.
2 A copy of the endoscopy report detailing the procedure, findings and any specific aftercare should be filed in the patient's notes.
3 Unless otherwise stated, patients may eat and drink once they are no longer drowsy and their gag reflex has returned.

What to look out for

It is important to be able to recognise adverse events following endoscopy on the ward.

The most common symptom associated with perforation is pain at the site. Cervical perforation of the oesophagus may lead to neck pain, dysphagia and hoarseness with subcutaneous emphysema. Intra-thoracic and abdominal perforations may result in chest or abdominal pain, guarding, rebound tenderness and abdominal distension.

Changes in the patient's observations (pulse, blood pressure or oxygen saturation) may all indicate that an adverse event has occurred. Monitor closely for signs of haemodynamic instability.

Delayed signs of perforation may also include fever, rising inflammatory markers and unusual radiographic features.

Management of perforation

1 Assess the patient's airway, breathing and circulation (ABC) first, as with any sick patient.
2 Get senior help. A gastrointestinal surgeon should assess the patient urgently.
3 As soon as the patient is haemodynamically stable, perform a plain erect CXR and abdominal film.
4 If there is no air on plain radiology, an abdominal CT scan may be recommended. This is a more sensitive test for pneumoperitoneum.
5 If there is evidence of free air, a contrast enema using water-soluble contrast may be indicated to differentiate between a free perforation and a localised sealed-off breach. This will affect decisions as to whether to adopt a conservative or surgical approach to management.

Lower GI endoscopy/colonoscopy

This is an examination of the colon using a fibre-optic endoscope that is introduced through the anus. The procedure is performed under light sedation. Diagnostic colonoscopy is indicated to investigate a change in bowel habit, iron-deficiency anaemia, weight loss or rectal bleeding, and to monitor inflammatory bowel disease (IBD). Therapeutic colonoscopy is used to treat any pathology that is found (e.g. to dilate strictures or remove polyps). As with upper GI endoscopy, many colonoscopies are performed as day-case outpatient procedures by gastroenterologists or lower GI surgeons. Junior doctors will be expected to know about the preparation of patients for colonoscopy, and their aftercare.

Colonoscopy is contraindicated in patients with a history of recent myocardial infarction (within the last 6 weeks), perforation of an abdominal viscus (when the insufflation with air may worsen faecal contamination of the peritoneal cavity), toxic fulminant colitis and severe un-reversed coagulopathy.

Complications of colonoscopy include perforation, bleeding, the introduction of infection, and respiratory depression secondary to sedation. Complications may be recognised immediately or may be delayed, and the risks are increased in frail, elderly patients and patients with a history of previous abdominal surgery, and those undergoing therapeutic procedures.

Prepare the patient

- Check the FBC, clotting and platelet count prior to the procedure. Guidelines suggest that it is safe to perform gastroscopy and biopsy if the platelet count is $> 70 \times 10^9$/l and the INR is < 1.5.
- Thorough bowel preparation prior to colonoscopy is a critical first step in ensuring a technically adequate study. Even small amounts of retained faecal matter can obscure the distal lens of the endoscope. Endoscopy units have different regimens, and it is therefore advisable that you discuss this with your endoscopy unit.
- Daily medications with small sips of water are allowed on the morning of colonoscopy. Patients at particular risk from dehydration, such as the elderly, should be commenced on maintenance IV fluids (e.g. 1 litre of 0.9% sodium chloride over 8–10 hours).
- Iron compounds should be discontinued 1 week before the procedure. Aspirin and aspirin-containing products should be stopped 5 days before the procedure to minimise the risk of bleeding (e.g. from polypectomy). This must be discussed with your consultant and the endoscopy department when the patient is listed, as failure to comply with endoscopy guidelines may result in a test being cancelled.
- The endoscopy department nurse in charge should be informed about any diabetic patients before the procedure so that these patients can be placed first on the list. Patients who are taking oral hypoglycaemic agents should omit their morning dose.
- Patients with metallic cardiac valve replacements will pose significant challenges with regard to anticoagulation, and must be discussed with your seniors.

Aftercare

1 Following endoscopy, patients will be transferred to a recovery area in the department for observation.
2 A copy of the endoscopy report detailing the procedure, findings and any specific aftercare should be filed in the patient's notes.
3 Unless otherwise stated, patients may eat and drink once they are no longer drowsy.

What to look out for

As with gastroscopy, it is important to be able to recognise immediate and delayed adverse events on the ward. Perforation is the chief concern, and abdominal pain with evidence of peritonism is the main symptom.

Close attention must be paid to the patient's observations following endoscopy to monitor for evidence of haemodynamic instability or of bacteraemia.

Abdominal X-ray (AXR)

Plain films of the abdomen are used primarily to assess for calcification and intestinal dilatation, perforation or obstruction. They are often used as an initial investigation, as they are quick to perform and easily available. Patients are required to lie flat or at a slight angle, and to stand for an erect film. Abdominal radiography is a non-invasive investigation. It exposes the patient to ionising radiation, and the radiation dose is equivalent to 50 anterior chest X-rays. Careful consideration should therefore be given to the decision to request it, and it is particularly unsuitable for pregnant women.

Approach to viewing films

1 Ensure that you have the correct films for the correct patient. Check the name, date of birth, sex and hospital number. Note any previous films available, as these can be used as a comparison.
2 Identify the projection of the film (most are AP) and the view taken (supine, erect or lateral decubitus). Unless specifically labelled, the film is assumed to be supine.
3 Four densities can be recognised on a film, namely black for gas, white for calcified structures, grey representing soft tissues, and darker grey for fat. Metallic objects are seen as an intense bright white.
4 Comment on the exposure. If the spine is visible, most structures to be seen will be visible. Areas of overexposure (dark areas) should be viewed with a bright light.
5 Comment on the area covered. An abdominal film should include the lower anterior ribs.
6 Note any artefacts (e.g. metallic objects, piercings, IUDs, clips from surgery).
7 Note the presence of intraluminal gas and its distribution. A gastric air bubble in the left upper quadrant is a normal finding. Gas may also be noted throughout the bowel.
8 Note the presence of extraluminal gas. Gas outside the bowel lumen is abnormal and indicates perforation of a viscus. Free air in the peritoneal

cavity is called a pneumoperitoneum. Gas in the biliary tree may be a normal finding after ERCP and sphincterotomy or biliary surgery.

9 Comment on the hollow organs that are visible.

- Small bowel may be seen. This should be less than 3 cm in diameter and lie centrally in the abdomen. Valvulae conniventes may be noted that cross the entire lumen. Dilated loops of bowel suggest obstruction or inflammation.
- Large bowel should lie at the periphery of the film. A normal colon should measure less than 5 cm in diameter. It can be differentiated from large bowel by haustra that cross only part of the bowel.

10 Consider the solid organs.

- Most solid organs are not visible on the plain AXR.
- The liver shadow may be recognised by the absence of bowel in the right upper quadrant. The kidneys may be noted as a shadow between T12 and L2, and the left kidney lies higher than the right one. The psoas muscles may be recognised as lines on either side of the lumbar spine extending to the lesser trochanter of the femur.
- Look for the presence of calcification. This may be normal in the costal cartilages and mesenteric lymph nodes. Abnormal calcification may indicate pathology in the pancreas, gallbladder (porcelain gallbladder), blood vessels and kidneys.
- Approximately 10–20% of gallstones are visible on plain AXR.
- Approximately 5% of renal calculi are visible. Look carefully at the pelvi-ureteric junction, the brim of the pelvis, and the vesico-ureteric junction for evidence of this.

11 Comment on the bones that are visible.

- The ribcage, lumbar spine, pelvis, sacrum and sacro-iliac joints may all be visible. Note the general bone density, presence of fractures, loss of joint space and cortical outlines.

Abdominal ultrasound (US)

Abdominal US obtains images of internal organs by sending high-frequency sound waves into the body. The reflected sound wave echoes are recorded and displayed as a real-time, visual image. US can therefore demonstrate blood flow and show movement of tissues.

US is the initial imaging modality of choice in patients with possible appendicitis, cholecystitis and renal or pelvic inflammatory disease. No ionising radiation (e.g. X-rays) is involved, so it is safe in pregnancy. The patient is required to lie flat or at a slight angle for the duration of the test (about 30 minutes). US is not suitable for patients who have recently had a barium enema, as retained barium may interfere with the quality of the test.

When the liver, gallbladder, spleen and pancreas are being imaged, the patient should be nil by mouth for 8–12 hours before the procedure. For renal ultrasound, the patient should be nil by mouth for 8–12 hours before the procedure, and about an hour before the test they will be required to drink four to six glasses of liquid to ensure that their bladder is full.

The abdominal computed tomography (CT) scan

CT scan images are created using a beam of X-rays that are recognised by a radiation detector. A computer then converts the CT scan into a three-dimensional image which can be viewed in 'slices.' It is an excellent method for visualising intra-abdominal solid organs and blood vessels.

A CT scan will expose the patient to ionising radiation, so its use must be carefully considered, particularly in the case of pregnant women. The patient must be able to lie flat on their back for the duration of the scan (about 20 minutes).

Depending on the indication, CT scans may be performed with or without contrast. Intravenous contrast is used to help to highlight blood vessels and to enhance the tissue structure of various organs, such as the brain, spine, liver and kidneys. Oral contrast is often used to enhance CT images of the abdomen and pelvis. Contrast studies must be discussed with a more senior doctor before requesting. Occasionally obstructions perforate, and contrast would be contraindicated.

It is important to check whether the patient has any allergies, particularly to contrast. In addition, patients with renal impairment are at greater risk if contrast agents are used. This situation can be avoided by ensuring that these patients are hydrated prior to the procedure (IV if NBM), avoiding the use of nephrotoxic agents, omitting metformin 48 hours before and after the procedure, and using N-acetyl cysteine (NAC) if required (e.g. 600 mg NAC by mouth twice a day). Discuss all patients with renal impairment with the radiology department before the procedure. Contrast use may be withheld if the creatinine level is > 150 µmol/l.

Further reading

- Longmore M, Wilkinson I, Turmezei T et al., eds. *Oxford Handbook of Clinical Medicine*, 7th edn. Oxford: Oxford University Press; 2009.
- Veitch AM, Baglin TP, Gershlick AH et al. Guidelines for the management of anticoagulant and antiplatelet therapy in patients undergoing endoscopic procedures. *Gut* 2008; **57**: 1322–9.
- Allison MC, Sandoe JAT, Tighe R et al. Antibiotic prophylaxis in gastrointestinal endoscopy. *Gut* 2010; **59**: 1300.

- Green J. *Complications of Gastrointestinal Endoscopy*. London: British Society of Gastroenterology; 2006.
- Endoscopy Section Committee of the British Society of Gastroenterology. *Safety and Sedation during Endoscopic Procedures*. London: British Society of Gastroenterology; 2003.
- Runyon BA, Montano AA, Akriviadis EA *et al.* The serum-ascites albumin gradient is superior to the exudate-transudate concept in the differential diagnosis of ascites. *Annals of Internal Medicine* 1992; **117:** 215–20.

4

Acute abdominal pain

Acute abdominal pain is defined as the onset of severe abdominal pain within the preceding 24 hours. In acute abdominal pain it may be difficult to make a diagnosis from the history and examination alone, and the use of imaging such as abdominal contrast-enhanced computed tomography (CT) and ultrasound scan (USS) are vital.

It is of primary importance in cases of abdominal pain to identify a 'surgical abdomen.' This is an acute intra-abdominal condition of abrupt onset, usually associated with pain due to inflammation, perforation, obstruction, infarction or rupture of abdominal organs, and usually requiring emergency intervention. It may be detected by the presence of pain, rebound tenderness, guarding and absent bowel sounds.

A ruptured ectopic pregnancy must be excluded as a first-line investigation for all female patients of childbearing age who present with abdominal pain. Abdominal pain in the elderly is of particular concern, as these patients may present late with vague symptoms, and signs of infection may be masked.

Aetiology
It is useful to categorise abdominal pain into three types:
1 **Visceral pain** is experienced when an abdominal viscus is stimulated. It may be experienced as dull, diffuse pain which is poorly localised to the midline, as innervation to most viscera is multi-segmental, and multiple viscera often converge on the same spinal neurons.
2 **Parietal pain** is experienced when the parietal peritoneum is stimulated. This pain often overlies the site of injury/inflammation and is sharp in nature. It is commonly made worse by coughing, straining and movement.
3 **Referred pain** is experienced at a site distant to the injury. The site of pain

is supplied by the same nerve root as the organ involved (e.g. pancreatic pain may radiate to the mid-back).

In abdominal pain it is useful to consider potential diagnoses by quadrant or region during the examination (*see* Figure 4.1). It must be remembered that any condition may present with generalised abdominal pain or with referred pain from other regions.

(a)   (b)

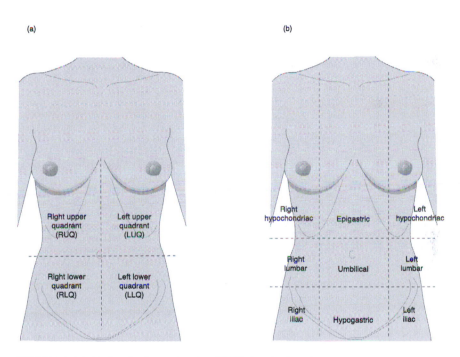

FIGURE 4.1 (a) Abdominal quadrants. (b) Abdominal regions.

Table 4.1 Common causes of abdominal pain by quadrant

Right upper quadrant	Biliary colic
	Cholangitis
	Cholecystitis
	Pancreatitis
	Liver disease
Left upper quadrant	Gastritis
	Peptic ulcer
	Splenomegaly

(*continued*)

Right lower quadrant	Renal colic
	Rupture (ovarian cyst, ectopic pregnancy, aortic aneurysm)
	Urinary tract infection
	Pyelonephritis
	Appendicitis
	Torsion
	Mesenteric adenitis
	Mesenteric infarction
	Volvulus (rotation of the gut on its mesenteric axis usually occurs at the level of the sigmoid, caecum or stomach)
	Pelvic inflammatory disease (PID)
	Diverticulitis
Left lower quadrant	Renal colic
	Rupture (ovarian cysts, ectopic pregnancy, aortic aneurysm)
	Torsion
	Urinary tract infection
	Pyelonephritis
	Diverticulitis
	Mesenteric adenitis
	Mesenteric infarction
	Volvulus (rotation of the gut on its mesenteric axis usually occurs at the level of the sigmoid, caecum or stomach)
	Pelvic inflammatory disease (PID)
Diffuse abdominal pain	Constipation
	Urinary retention
	Perforated viscus
	Ileus
	Mechanical obstruction

Adapted from the Merck Manuals Online Medical Library website. www.merckmanuals.com/professional/sec02/ch011/ch011b.html Acute abdominal pain. Last full revision September 2007 by Parswa Ansari.

Common causes of abdominal pain include the following:
- constipation
- biliary tract disease
- diverticulitis
- appendicitis

- UTI
- bowel obstruction
- mesenteric ischaemia
- peptic ulcer disease.

Biliary tract disease

Biliary tract disease is a common cause of abdominal pain. In the elderly it accounts for more than 25% of patients who present with abdominal pain and require hospitalisation.

Patients may present with fever, right upper quadrant pain, a raised white cell count (WCC) and inflammatory markers, and deranged liver function tests (predominantly an obstructive picture). A USS of the hepatobiliary system is the investigation of choice, looking for evidence of a dilated CBD and intrahepatic ducts, gallstones and an inflamed gallbladder.

Diverticulae

Diverticulae are out-pouchings of the mucosa and sub-mucosa through the wall of the bowel. They are very common, and the frequency of occurrence increases with age. The majority of patients will experience no complications. However, diverticulitis occurs when diverticulae become obstructed by faecal matter. This may present as a fever, a raised WCC and a mass (often in the left lower quadrant).

The Hinchey classification system is a useful way of categorising the complications of diverticulitis:

- Stage 1: small pericolic or mesenteric abscess.
- Stage 2: larger abscess extending into the pelvis.
- Stage 3: rupture of a diverticular abscess, leading to purulent peritonitis.
- Stage 4: faeculent peritonitis (rupture of a diverticulum that is not inflamed or obstructed, leading to the release of faecal material directly into the peritoneum).

CT is the investigation of choice in patients with suspected diverticulitis. Management consists of IV antibiotics and surgery for peritonitis, perforation, large abscesses, sepsis and failure to improve on medical management.

Appendicitis

This is inflammation of the appendix. It has a high mortality rate in the elderly, with half of all deaths occurring in patients over 60 years of age. Appendicitis can be a difficult diagnosis to make, as pain may not always localise to the right lower quadrant, and not all patients present with fever and a raised white cell count. CT is an excellent investigation in cases of suspected appendicitis, and management consists of surgery.

The Alvarado score predicts the likelihood of appendicitis in the presence of certain signs and symptoms.

TABLE 4.2 Alvarado scoring system

SYMPTOM	SCORE
Migration of pain	1
Anorexia	1
Raised temperature (>37.3 °C)	1
Rebound pain	1
Tenderness in the right iliac fossa	2
Nausea, vomiting	1
Differential white blood cell count >75% neutrophils	1
Elevated white cell count	2
Total	10

A score of 9 or 10 indicates very probable acute appendicitis.
A score of 7 or 8 indicates probable appendicitis.
A score of 5 or 6 is suggestive of appendicitis.

Mesenteric ischaemia (abdominal angina)

This is a more uncommon cause of abdominal pain, but it has a high mortality rate. Affected patients often have a history of smoking, hyperlipidaemia, diabetes or peripheral arterial disease. Mesenteric ischaemia may be precipitated by a meal, and pain usually follows 30–90 minutes post-prandially.

It has three possible causes:
1 thrombotic (arterial thrombus accounts for one-third of cases)
2 non-occlusive (often due to severe and prolonged intestinal vasoconstriction, which may be secondary to severe sepsis/illness)
3 embolic (emboli to mesenteric arteries).

Intestinal obstruction

Either the small or large intestine may become obstructed, and it can be a challenge to differentiate between the two clinically. Obstruction may be mechanical or caused by an ileus (non-mechanical cause, e.g. electrolyte disturbances and certain medications). Patients may present with abdominal pain, abdominal distension and nausea, with associated constipation, vomiting and absent bowel sounds.

Diagnosis is with an abdominal X-ray (AXR) and contrast studies. The patient should be kept nil by mouth, with an NG tube in place on free drainage. Underlying electrolyte abnormalities should be corrected and urgent surgical review undertaken.

Peptic ulcer disease (PUD)

Peptic ulcers are defects in the GI mucosa, often caused by *Helicobacter pylori* infection or the use of aspirin or non-steroidal anti-inflammatory drugs (NSAIDs). The term PUD incorporates both gastric and duodenal ulcers. The first evidence of disease may be GI bleeding with or without abdominal pain.

Complications of PUD include perforation, bleeding and the formation of localised strictures. These are managed with diagnostic (and possibly also therapeutic) endoscopy, surgery and the use of gastric acid suppressants.

Urinary tract infection (UTI)

UTI is a common cause of abdominal pain, and is defined as the presence of bacteria in the urine in addition to the presence of symptoms (e.g. dysuria, frequency and urgency). Infections of the urinary tract may be diagnosed by urinalysis (e.g. urine dipstick and midstream specimen of urine).

Pyelonephritis may develop as a complication of UTIs. This is an infection of the renal parenchyma, and it may present with urinary symptoms, fever and raised inflammatory markers. It is a potentially serious infection that requires urgent treatment.

Clinical presentation

History

A full medical history is required in all patients who present with abdominal pain. It is important to enquire about the following:

- **History of the pain:** site, onset, radiation, quality, duration, exacerbating and relieving factors, as well as previous episodes of pain.
- **Vomiting:** frequency, presence of blood or foodstuff in the vomitus, and the relationship to food. Vomiting is an early symptom if there is an obstruction high up in the GI tract.
- **Urinary symptoms:** urinary frequency, dysuria, urgency and haematuria may occur in UTIs, pyelonephritis and renal colic.
- **Bowel habit:** constipation, diarrhoea, presence of rectal bleeding and passage of flatus.
- **Associated symptoms:** fever and rigors may point to infection as a cause.
- **Menstrual and sexual history:** last menstrual period (LMP) and the

possibility of pregnancy. Abnormal vaginal discharge may indicate pelvic inflammatory disease.

- **Medical history:** diabetes, ischaemic heart disease (which may point to mesenteric ischaemia as the cause).
- **Previous surgery:** this may suggest adhesions or strictures as the possible cause of pain.
- **Medication use:** over-the-counter medication, herbal supplements and recreational drugs.
- **Alcohol and smoking history:** pancreatitis may be alcohol-induced, and smoking may increase the risk of vascular complications (e.g. mesenteric infarction).

Infection may be masked in the elderly. Do not rely on fever or raised white cell count alone, and retain a high index of suspicion at all times.

Examination

Perform a full system examination, looking for evidence of the following:

- **General status** (e.g. the presence of pain, sepsis and shock): This may indicate the severity of the underlying condition and the condition of the patient.
- **Dehydration:** this may indicate vomiting or electrolyte disturbance.
- **Signs of sepsis** (e.g. cholecystitis, pancreatitis or peritonitis).
- **Abdominal distension:** this may be evidence of both mechanical and non-mechanical obstruction. If you are unsure whether distension is present, take serial measurements of abdominal girth (at the same place on the abdomen) each time the patient is examined.
- **Bowel sounds:** bowel sounds are traditionally absent in ileus, and high-pitched and tinkling in mechanical obstruction. A succussion splash may be heard in outflow tract obstruction (a splash-like sound that is heard during auscultation with or without a stethoscope when the abdomen of a patient with outflow obstruction is gently shaken from side to side).
- **Peritonism:** look for evidence of rebound tenderness (*see* Chapter 1), abdominal rigidity and voluntary guarding, which may indicate an inflammatory process of the abdominal peritoneum.
- **Renal angle tenderness:** this may be present in pyelonephritis.
- **Tender hepatomegaly:** this may be found in acute cases of jaundice.
- **Hernial orifices:** inspect for evidence of an incarcerated hernia.
- **Pulsatile masses and peripheral pulses:** look for evidence of an aortic aneurysm.
- **Rectal and pelvic examination:** a rectal examination is mandatory in patients with abdominal pain, in order to exclude constipation and

look for evidence of PR bleeding. A pelvic examination in women should usually be left to an expert, as it is a sensitive procedure, and interpretation of the findings requires experience.

- **Respiratory examination:** look for evidence of pneumonia, which may mimic abdominal pain.
- **Cardiovascular examination:** myocardial infarctions can present with abdominal pain, nausea and vomiting. Atrial fibrillation or ischaemia on an ECG is suggestive of mesenteric ischaemia as a cause of abdominal pain.

Initial Investigations

- **FBC.** Leucocytosis suggests infection (but WCC may be raised in any cause of abdominal pain), and anaemia may indicate occult bleeding or haemolysis. A reactive thrombocytosis may be present.
- **U&Es.** Dehydration and electrolyte abnormalities may occur secondary to vomiting. Both may also contribute to the development of ileus.
- **LFTs.** Derangement may suggest a hepatobiliary cause of pain.
- **Glucose.** Raised glucose levels may be the result of stress. However, a very high glucose level may indicate diabetic ketoacidosis or a hyperosmolar non-ketotic state as an atypical cause of pain.
- **Amylase.** Levels may be raised in many causes of abdominal pain. A rise in amylase levels to more than 4 times the normal limit is usually diagnostic of pancreatitis. Amylase levels are often not raised in patients with chronic pancreatitis.
- **CRP.** Levels may be raised in any cause of abdominal pain.
- **ABG.** Acidosis and raised lactate levels is an indication of the severity of the underlying illness, and are a poor prognostic feature.
- **Group and save.** This is important if the patient is bleeding or may require surgery.
- **Clotting.** This may be useful if there is suspected coagulopathy, chronic liver disease, or pre-operatively.
- **Urine dip and MC&S.** These are used to exclude UTI and pyelonephritis as the cause of pain.
- **Pregnancy test.** This must be performed in every female patient of childbearing age.
- **ECG.** A sinus tachycardia is common in the context of pain alone. However, it may help to exclude other atypical presentations, such as a myocardial infarction or pulmonary embolism.
- **Erect CXR.** Look for free air under the diaphragm in perforation. Pneumonia may also mimic abdominal pain and be picked up as consolidation or effusion on the CXR.

- **AXR.** Look for evidence of dilated loops of bowel, air in the biliary tree, and renal and biliary calculi.

Further investigations

Abdominal USS

This is the initial imaging of choice in patients with possible appendicitis, cholecystitis, or renal or pelvic inflammatory disease. Ultrasound is relatively inexpensive, and does not involve the use of ionising radiation. It is therefore safe to use in pregnancy. However, images may be difficult to obtain if the patient has a large amount of adipose tissue.

Abdominal CT

This is the initial imaging of choice in patients with pancreatitis or suspected abdominal aortic aneurysm. CT may also be beneficial in any situation that potentially requires surgery, as an aid to the planning of the procedure.

Undergoing a CT scan is likely to involve movement of the patient from a ward or Accident and Emergency setting to the radiology department. It is vital to ensure that the patient is stable enough to undergo transfer. On occasion medical staff will be required to accompany the patient for this investigation.

In cases of impaired renal function it is vital to discuss the patient with the radiology department, as the contrast that is used in imaging may worsen kidney disease. Also ensure that the patient does not have a history of previous allergic reactions to contrast media.

IVU/IVP

This can be useful in cases of suspected ureteric stones. A plain AXR is performed, followed by the administration of contrast. A repeat AXR is performed 30 minutes later, with the possibility of further ones at 30-minute intervals.

As contrast is used, it is important to check the patient's renal function and history of previous allergies to contrast before performing the procedure.

Management

The management of abdominal pain depends on its cause.

Medical management

Until imaging or other investigations have yielded a definitive diagnosis, general management principles should be followed.

In the initial stages these should follow the Airway, Breathing, Circulation, Disability, Exposure format, as with any sick patient.

- Obtain senior help early on:
  — medical registrar
  — surgical registrar.
- Manage airway and breathing first.
  — Give oxygen 60–100%.
  — Consider contacting an anaesthetist and asking them to assess the patient's airway if there is evidence of hypoxia or impaired consciousness.
- Circulation:
  — Good IV access is vital.
  — Site a large-bore cannula (14- to 16-gauge).
  — Take blood samples for FBC, U&Es, LFTs, amylase, glucose, clotting, and group and save (if there is evidence of shock or bleeding) when inserting the cannula.
  — IV fluid resuscitation is very important. Correction of electrolyte disturbance may facilitate the return of normal bowel function in pseudo-obstruction, and is important for optimising patients prior to surgery.
  — Consider inserting a urinary catheter to monitor urine output.
  — Attach a cardiac monitor and a pulse oximeter.
- Nasogastric tube placement to drain gastric contents may be appropriate if abdominal distension from obstruction is present.
- It is wise to keep the patient nil by mouth (NBM) until they have been seen by a surgeon.
- Arterial blood gases (ABGs) and lactate levels should be measured if there is hypoxia or shock.
- Perform a urine dip and send urine for MC&S.
- Seek the patient's consent for a pregnancy test.
- AXR with or without erect CXR should be performed if perforation is suspected.
- Regular observations are necessary.
- Obtain an urgent surgical opinion if there is any evidence of peritonism.
- Antibiotics should be given if infection is suspected (follow local trust guidelines).

Daily monitoring/investigation

1   Close observation of vital signs.
2   Fluid balance, including urine output and presence of vomitus.

3 Presence of abdominal distension – it may be appropriate to make daily repeat abdominal girth measurements.
4 Bowel movements and the passage of flatus should be recorded on a stool chart.
5 Perform an AXR and erect CXR on the day of admission, and repeat these urgently if the patient deteriorates.

Important tips

Surgeons
Discuss cases with the surgeons early in the patient's presentation. If medical causes of abdominal pain have been excluded, it is more appropriate for the patient to be managed under a surgical team.

Ensure that an erect CXR, AXR and routine bloods have been sent before making a surgical referral, unless the diagnosis is thought to be a surgical emergency (e.g. a leaking abdominal aortic aneurysm). Surgical emergencies should trigger prompt surgical referral and focus on stabilising the patient.

Obstetrics and gynaecology
It may be appropriate to discuss cases with O&G. Prior to referral, ensure that a pregnancy test has been carried out and the results noted.

Cannulae
Intravenous cannulae are a common source of infection in hospitals. Ensure that you change the cannula every 3 days, and inspect the cannula site daily for early signs of local infection. Write the date of insertion on the cannula dressing, and record this in the notes to avoid confusion.

Previous records
Review the patient's case notes, particularly for details of previous imaging or surgical procedures.

Information to have to hand for ward rounds
1 Up-to-date bloods, including FBC, U&Es, CRP, LFTs and amylase.
2 Urine dipstick result, including pregnancy test results.
3 The results of any imaging (e.g. USS, CT, IVU).
4 Up-to-date microbiology results if appropriate.
5 Observation chart for temperature and haemodynamic status.

Further reading

- Travis S, Ahmad T, Collier J *et al. Pocket Consultant Gastroenterology*, 3rd edn. Oxford: Wiley-Blackwell; 2005.
- Merck Manuals Online Medical Library website. www.merckmanuals.com/professional/sec02.html Acute abdominal pain. Last full revision September 2007 by Parswa Ansari.
- Longmore M, Wilkinson I, Turmezei T *et al.*, eds. *Oxford Handbook of Clinical Medicine*, 7th edn. Oxford: Oxford University Press; 2009.
- McNally PR. *GI/Liver Secrets Plus*, 4th edn. Philadelphia, PA: Mosby; 2010.

5

Acute gastrointestinal haemorrhage

Acute gastrointestinal haemorrhage is bleeding from the GI tract, which may occur at any point in the GI tract and is classified as originating from an upper GI or lower GI source. It may be an occult or incidental finding, or it may present with massive blood loss and haemodynamic instability. GI bleeds have an incidence of approximately 90 per 100 000 adults per year. The incidence increases with age, and they are twice as common in men as in women.

It is vital to swiftly identify haemodynamically unstable patients, those at risk of further re-bleeding, and those with conditions that have a high morbidity and mortality rate.

Epidemiology/aetiology

Upper GI bleeding (UGIB)

This is bleeding that occurs proximal to the ligament of Treitz, which connects the duodenum to the diaphragm and is the landmark of the duodenojejeunal junction. It may present as haematemesis, 'coffee-ground vomiting' and/or melaena. Very brisk upper GI bleeding may present as fresh blood per rectum.

UGIB represents 80% of all GI bleeds, and the overall mortality rate is 10% (a total of 5000 deaths annually in the UK). Both incidence and mortality increase with age, and 45% of GI bleeds occur in those over 60 years of age. Death in elderly patients with a UGIB is frequently due to exacerbation of comorbid conditions. UGIB is twice as common in men, and is more prevalent among the lower socio-economic classes. There may be a history of aspirin or NSAID use.

Patients with UGIB may present with haematemesis (50% of cases), melaena (30%), or haematemesis and melaena (20%), or UGIB may be an occult finding (e.g. in the investigation of anaemia).

The most common causes of UGIB include the following:[1]

- **Duodenal ulcers (35%):** these are strongly associated with *Helicobacter pylori* infection (leading to inflammation of the mucosa and degradation of the protective mucus barrier, resulting in ulcer formation).
- **Gastric ulcers (20%):** these may be induced by *H. pylori*, aspirin or NSAIDs disrupting the mucosal response to acid.
- **Gastroduodenal erosions (8–15%):** these may be linked to gastro-oesophageal reflux, infection, medications, the ingestion of caustic substances, or radiation.
- **Mallory–Weiss syndrome (15%):** this is bleeding from lacerations of the mucosa at the gastro-oesophageal junction, gastric cardia, or distal oesophagus. It may be caused by forceful vomiting.
- **Varices (15%):** these are collateral veins that develop as a result of obstruction to hepatic portal vein flow, with a consequent rise in portal venous pressure leading to portal gastropathy.

UGIB may be arterial (e.g. peptic ulcer disease) or venous (e.g. telangiectasia) in origin. Variceal bleeding is a particularly serious type of upper GI bleed, with a high re-bleed and mortality rate (up to 8% of patients within 48 hours). A variceal bleed must be suspected if a patient is known to have liver disease, has a history of heavy alcohol consumption, or has stigmata of chronic liver disease, such as ascites, jaundice, spider naevi, abnormal liver function tests or deranged clotting.

BOX 5.1 Risk factors for increased mortality, re-bleeding, need for surgery or endoscopy in (non-variceal) UGIB, according to Scottish Intercollegiate Guidelines Network (SIGN) guidance

- Increasing age
- Comorbidity
- Liver disease
- Inpatients
- Presence of shock
- Continued bleeding after admission
- Haematemesis
- Haematochezia
- Elevated blood urea

It is important to identify at an early stage those patients who may be suffering from a variceal bleed, who are haemodynamically unstable, or who are at high risk of re-bleeding or significant comorbidity, as these patients have a higher mortality rate than the general population (*see* Box 5.1).

Scoring tools are available that can be used to predict mortality and morbidity in UGIB. The Rockall score is a tool that can help to stratify patients at risk of death and re-bleeding (*see* Table 5.1). It is calculated prior to endoscopy and then modified once the patient has undergone endoscopy.

TABLE 5.1 The Rockall risk assessment score

VARIABLE	SCORE			
	0	1	2	3
Age (years)	<60	60–79	≥80	–
Shock (BP and pulse)	>100 mmHg <100 bpm	>100 mmHg >100 bpm	<100 mmHg >100 bpm	–
Comorbidity	None	–	Cardiac disease, any other major comorbidity	Renal failure, liver failure, disseminated malignancy
Endoscopic diagnosis	Mallory–Weiss tear, no lesion	All other diagnoses	Malignancy of the upper GI tract	–
Major SRH	None, or dark spots	–	Blood in the upper GI tract, adherent clot or spurting vessel	–

BP, blood pressure; GI, gastrointestinal; SRH, stigmata of recent haemorrhage.

Table 5.2 shows the re-bleed and mortality risk as calculated by the Rockall score.

TABLE 5.2 Re-bleed and mortality risk according to Rockall score

RISK SCORE	PREDICTED RE-BLEED RISK (%)	PREDICTED MORTALITY RISK (%)
0	5	0
1	3	0
2	5	0
3	11	3
4	14	5
5	24	11
6	33	17

Adapted from Rockall TA, Logan RFA, Devlin HB *et al.*[2]

Lower GI bleeding

Lower GI haemorrhage is bleeding distal to the ligament of Treitz. It includes bleeding from both the small bowel and the colon. It usually presents with fresh blood per rectum.

Acute lower tract haemorrhage accounts for approximately 20% of all GI bleeds. They are more common in men, and there may be a history of aspirin or NSAID use. Patients may present with fresh red blood per rectum (although you will need to consider whether this could be from a brisk upper GI source), or with dark blood with clots or mixed with faeces. Lower GI bleeds have a mortality rate of approximately 4%.

Common causes of lower GI bleeding include the following:

- **Diverticulae (55%):** out-pouchings of colonic submucosa and mucosa through weakened muscle layers; these typically occur in the sigmoid colon.
- **Haemorrhoids (< 10%):** arterio-venous channels and connective tissue in the rectum that become inflamed.
- **Inflammatory bowel disease of the GI mucosa.**

Clinical presentation

Targeted history for lower GI bleeding:

- onset of bleeding
- type of blood (fresh, dark with clots)
- pain during defecation
- blood mixed with stool, on pan and on toilet paper
- frequency of bleeding
- association with defecation
- change in bowel habit
- weight loss and/or abdominal pain
- medical history
- drug history (aspirin and other NSAIDs, anti-platelets and anticoagulants).

Targeted history for upper GI bleeding:

- number of episodes of vomiting
- presence of any blood/coffee grounds
- melaena
- fresh red blood per rectum
- estimate of blood loss (e.g. a cupful), although this should not be regarded as particularly precise
- episodes of retching or forceful vomiting prior to the appearance of blood in vomitus raises the suspicion of a Mallory–Weiss tear

- previous episodes of UGIB
- use of iron tablets
- use of beta-blockers or calcium-channel blockers (which may suppress a sympathetic cardiovascular response to hypovolaemia)
- symptoms of postural hypotension
- history of alcohol misuse
- known liver disease.

It is important to document the presence or absence of the following features in your examination:
- Age – mortality and morbidity increase with age.
- Comorbidity – the presence of ischaemic heart disease, renal failure and malignancy increase a patient's morbidity and mortality.
- Stigmata of chronic liver disease (e.g. ascites, caput medusa or gynaecomastia), which may indicate that varices are a cause of bleeding and suggest an underlying coagulopathy.
- Features suggestive of malignancy (e.g. weight loss, dysphagia).
- It is vital to note and document the patient's haemodynamic status. The degree of shock should be estimated (*see* Table 5.3).
- Always perform a rectal examination. Document the presence or absence of normal stool, fresh blood or melaena.
- Fresh blood per rectum is unlikely to be from an upper GI source unless there has been brisk bleeding associated with haemodynamic changes.

TABLE 5.3 Clinical signs of haemorrhagic shock

	CLASS 1	CLASS 2	CLASS 3	CLASS 4
Blood loss Volume in adult (ml)	< 750	750–1499	1500–2000	> 2000
Blood loss (as % of circulating blood volume)	< 15	15–29	30–40	> 40
Pulse rate (beats/min)	< 100	> 100	> 120	> 140
Blood pressure	Normal	Decreased	Decreased	Decreased
Capillary refill	Normal	Normal	Increased	Absent
Urine output (ml/hour)	> 30	20–30	5–19	< 5
Respiratory rate (breaths/min)	14–19	20–29	30–40	> 35
Mental state	Normal	Anxious	Confused	Lethargic

Adapted from Baskett PJF.[3]

Initial investigations

- **FBC.** Normocytic anaemia in the case of an acute bleed. Microcytic anaemia may suggest chronic bleeding. Thrombocytopenia may coexist with chronic liver disease.
- **U&Es.** Renal function may be deranged secondary to intravascular depletion. A disproportionately high urea to creatinine ratio suggests that there is a high protein load in the gut from fresh blood.
- **LFTs.** These may be abnormal in chronic liver disease. Hypoalbuminaemia may reflect poor synthetic liver function.
- **Coagulation screen.** This may be deranged in chronic liver disease with a prolonged PT/INR.
- **ECG.** This may demonstrate ischaemic changes in cases of severe hypovolaemia or pre-existing heart disease.
- **CXR.** A baseline CXR is useful to look for evidence of aspiration, particularly if the patient has lost consciousness and vomited. It may also help to rule out a GI tract perforation with free air under the hemi-diaphragm.
- **Group and save.** This must be done in the case of every GI bleed. Cross-match 6 units of whole blood if there is shock or signs of a major bleed, and 4 units in smaller bleeds. Contact the transfusion laboratory and discuss your needs with them.
- **ABGs.** These are required if there is evidence of hypoxia or shock.

Further investigations

Oesophagogastroduodenoscopy

The timing of oesophagogastroduodenoscopy (OGD) is dependent on the clinical status of the patient. Emergency endoscopy (immediate and/ or out of hours) is performed in massive bleeds, in patients with known variceal bleeds, and in those who continue to bleed or re-bleed following endoscopy. Other patients will usually have an endoscopy urgently (within 24–48 hours), and very stable patients may be sent home for outpatient endoscopy. These decisions are made on the basis of the patient's clinical presentation, comorbidity, history and Rockall score.

Colonoscopy

This procedure can diagnose up to 90% of colonic bleeds.

Mesenteric angiography

This is a particularly valuable technique for identifying the bleeding source in angiodysplasia (a vascular malformation). It is both a diagnostic and therapeutic procedure.

Technetium-99m-labelled red cell scintigraphy

This involves labelling the patient's own red cells with a radionuclide in order to identify the source of bleeding. It is traditionally used when other modalities have failed.

In the case of small bowel bleeds, there are several other diagnostic and therapeutic procedures available. These are summarised below.

Video capsule endoscopy

This is a small pill-sized endoscope that is swallowed and passes through the GI tract. This procedure will provide images of the gut, but does not take samples for histology.

Double-balloon endoscopy

This allows the whole bowel to be visualised through the use of a modified enteroscope.

Barium small bowel follow-through

The patient swallows contrast medium, which appears white on X-rays. This procedure allows visualisation of the gross anatomy of the small bowel.

Conventional and magnetic resonance enteroclysis

Radio contrast is introduced through a tube from the nose to the duodenum. The small bowel is distended by contrast, and CT or MRI images are obtained.

Management

In the context of an acute GI bleed the patient may or may not be fasted. Although this is unlikely to affect the management, it is important to document the time when the patient last ate and drank, and to inform the anaesthetist of this. The patient will need to provide written consent to endoscopic investigation and management unless they are unable to do so (e.g. because they are obtunded).

Medical management

In the initial stages this should follow the ABCDE format (as with any sick patient).
- Obtain senior help early on:
  — medical registrar
  — on-call gastroenterology registrar.
- Manage airway and breathing first.
  — Give 60–100% oxygen.

- — Consider contacting an anaesthetist to assess the patient's airway if there is evidence of hypoxia, torrential bleeding or impaired consciousness. These patients may need intubation prior to endoscopy, in order to protect their airway and reduce the risk of aspiration.
- Circulation:
  - — Good IV access is vital.
  - — Site at least two large-bore cannulas (14- to 16-gauge).
  - — Patients who are at risk of exsanguination may require central access (e.g. via internal jugular vein).
  - — Fluid resuscitation – either colloid or crystalloid solutions may be used to achieve volume restoration prior to administering blood products.
  - — As part of monitoring the circulation, a urinary catheter should be inserted and hourly urine output measurements obtained.
- All patients must have a group and save.
  - — In any major bleed, cross-match 6 units of blood.
  - — Blood transfusion is required when estimated blood loss is greater than 30% of the circulating blood volume (1500 ml in an adult).
  - — Give unmatched O Rhesus-negative blood in an extreme emergency.
  - — Always keep 2 units of blood in reserve.
- Patients with chronic liver disease and those with deranged clotting or a low platelet count will need early discussion with a haematologist and consideration of blood product replacement. They may require:
  - — FFP if the PT is > 20s and/or APTT is > 48s (give 10–15 ml/kg of FFP, or 4 units)
  - — cryoprecipitate if the fibrinogen level is < 1 g/l (give 1–1.5 packs/10 kg body weight)
  - — platelets if the count is < 50 × 10^9/l.
- Patients should be fasted prior to endoscopy unless there is a life-threatening haemorrhage and endoscopy has to be performed urgently. Otherwise they should remain fasted from midnight the day before. Ensure that supplemental IV fluids are prescribed to prevent dehydration.
- A stool chart should be used to document the amount, colour and frequency of bowel movements.

Upper GI bleeding
- A Rockall score should be calculated for all patients.
- Patients with a Rockall score of 0 may be considered for non-admission or early discharge with outpatient follow-up (this decision should only be made by a senior).

- In patients with an initial (pre-endoscopic) Rockall score of > 0, endoscopy is recommended for a full assessment of bleeding risk.
- Patients with a post-endoscopic score of < 3 have a low risk of re-bleeding or death, and should be considered for early discharge and outpatient follow-up.
- Patients with a GI bleed should be managed in a dedicated GI bleed unit.
- Proton pump inhibitors (PPIs) should not be used prior to diagnosis by endoscopy. You may find that their use prior to endoscopy differs in clinical practice.
- High-dose PPIs (e.g. pantoprazole 80 mg bolus followed by 8 mg/hour infusion over 72 hours) should be used in patients with major peptic ulcer bleeding following endoscopy.

Variceal bleeding

Much of the general management is the same as that of an upper GI bleed, following the ABCDE format of assessment.
- Obtain senior help early on:
  — duty medical registrar
  — duty gastroenterology registrar
  — duty haematology registrar
  — duty anaesthetist.
- Airway and breathing:
  — Give 60–100% oxygen, and consider using an ET tube if there is torrential bleeding or impaired consciousness.
- Secure circulatory access:
  — Site two large-bore cannulas.
- Circulation.
  — Correct hypovolaemia.
  — Begin rapid colloid infusion to maintain systolic blood pressure > 90 mmHg (e.g. Gelofusine 500 ml at once).
  — Consider giving O Rhesus-negative blood if the patient is in extremis.
- Give terlipressin to reduce portal pressure by splanchnic vasoconstriction prior to endoscopy (e.g. 2 mg IV followed by 1–2 mg every 4–6 hours until bleeding is controlled, and then post-endoscopy for up to 72 hours).
- Arrange an urgent endoscopy. This will take place once the patient is haemodynamically stable.
- A gastroenterology registrar or consultant may consider using a Sengstaken–Blakemore tube to control life-threatening variceal bleeding acutely if this is uncontrolled by endoscopy.

- Transjugular intrahepatic portosystemic shunting may be used to treat uncontrolled variceal bleeding.
- In patients with chronic liver disease and variceal bleeding, give prophylactic antibiotics (e.g. ciprofloxacin IV for 7–10 days) (always consult your local guidelines).

Lower GI bleeding
- The cause and site of massive lower GI haemorrhage should be determined following the early use of colonoscopy and CT, CT angiography or digital subtraction angiography (DSA).
- Nuclear scintigraphy (the use of radionuclides) should be considered to aid the localisation of bleeding in patients with significant recent haemorrhage.
- In patients with massive lower GI haemorrhage, colonoscopic haemostasis is an effective means of controlling haemorrhage from active diverticular bleeding and post-polypectomy bleeding, when appropriately skilled expertise is available.
- In patients with massive lower GI haemorrhage, if colonoscopy fails to define the site of bleeding and control haemorrhage, angiographic transarterial embolisation is recommended as an effective means of controlling haemorrhage.
- Localised segmental intestinal resection or subtotal colectomy is recommended for the management of colonic haemorrhage that is uncontrolled by other techniques.

Surgical management
Indications for surgical management in patients with GI bleeding are as follows:
- severe life-threatening haemorrhage that is not responsive to resuscitative efforts
- failure of both medical therapy and endoscopic therapy, with persistent recurrent bleeding
- a coexisting reason for surgery, such as perforation, obstruction or malignancy
- prolonged bleeding with loss of 50% or more of the patient's blood volume.

Angiographic embolisation is an option for patients who are poor candidates for surgery.

Daily monitoring/investigations

1   Close observation of vital signs, including temperature, blood pressure, pulse, respiratory rate and saturations.
2   Daily review of clinical condition, stool charts, and the presence of haematemesis or melaena.
3   Daily examination, looking specifically for evidence of bleeding, and haemodynamic and hydration status.
4   Daily bloods, including FBC and U&Es. Clotting should be repeated weekly if the results are abnormal initially.

Important tips

Rockall score

Estimation of the patient's Rockall score is a tool that can help to stratify patients at risk of death and re-bleeding. It is calculated before and after endoscopy.

Endoscopy request forms

When booking an endoscopy, always document the patient's Rockall score, their haemodynamic status, their most recent haemoglobin, platelets and coagulation screen, any recent use of anticoagulant/antiplatelet drugs and any comorbidity. If possible, discuss the case with the on-call gastroenterology registrar or consultant. Always put your name and bleep number on the form, as this will enable the endoscopy department to contact you easily if they have any questions.

Diabetic patients

Patients on insulin should commence a sliding scale prior to endoscopy. Those on oral hypoglycaemic agents should have their medications withheld and be discussed with the endoscopy department, who may place them first on the list.

Anticoagulant and antiplatelet drugs

In the event of elective endoscopy, ensure that anticoagulants such as warfarin and enoxaparin have been stopped if possible (otherwise discuss this with a gastroenterologist). Deranged clotting may need to be corrected. Antiplatelet agents such as aspirin and clopidogrel may also need to be stopped. In the case of patients with a history of recent cardiac intervention, discuss this with a cardiologist first.

Discharge care

It is useful to send the GP a copy of the patient's endoscopy result, post-endoscopy haemoglobin and hospital follow-up information. Patients should be advised to avoid alcohol, NSAIDS, antiplatelet agents and/or anticoagulants if appropriate. They should be provided with information about their diagnosis, and a management plan should be agreed.

Information to have to hand for ward rounds

1 Up-to-date bloods, including FBC, U&Es, LFTs and clotting.
2 Observation chart for haemodynamic status.
3 Stool chart for evidence of melaena.
4 Results of endoscopy, or the date when endoscopy is booked.

References

1 Travis S, Ahmad T, Collier J *et al. Pocket Consultant Gastroenterology*, 3rd edn. Oxford: Wiley-Blackwell; 2005.
2 Rockall TA, Logan RFA, Devlin HB *et al.* Selection of patients for early discharge or outpatient care after acute upper gastrointestinal haemorrhage. *Lancet* 1996; **347:** 1138–40.
3 Baskett PJF. ABC of major trauma. Management of hypovolaemic shock. *British Medical Journal* 1990; **300:** 1453–7.

Further reading

- Rockall TA, Logan RFA, Devlin HB *et al.* Selection of patients for early discharge or outpatient care after acute upper gastrointestinal haemorrhage. *Lancet* 1996; **347:** 1138–40.
- Travis S, Ahmad T, Collier J *et al. Pocket Consultant Gastroenterology*, 3rd edn. Oxford: Wiley-Blackwell; 2005.
- Scottish Intercollegiate Guidelines Network. *Management of Acute Upper and Lower GI Bleeding*. Guideline No. 105. Edinburgh: Scottish Intercollegiate Guidelines Network; 2008.
- Gutierrez G, Reines HD, and Wulf-Gutierrez ME. Clinical review: haemorrhagic shock. *Critical Care* 2004; **8:** 373–81.
- Rockall TA, Logan RFA, Devlin HB *et al.* Risk assessment after acute upper gastrointestinal haemorrhage. *Gut* 1996; **38:** 316–21.

6

Gastro-oesophageal reflux disease

Gastro-oesophageal reflux disease (GORD) can be simply defined as the reflux of gastric contents into the oesophagus, leading to oesophagitis and subsequent complications such as ulceration, stricture formation, Barrett's oesophagus and adenocarcinoma formation. It can be subdivided into reflux oesophagitis and non-erosive reflux disease.

Epidemiology

GORD is particularly common in Western populations, with an incidence of 5–10%. The incidence is significantly lower in the East Asian population, at around 5%. The vast majority of individuals will experience symptoms of acid reflux/indigestion at some stage in their lifetime. However, these symptoms often do not meet the diagnostic criteria of GORD.

Aetiology

Studies have demonstrated that increasing age and male gender are associated with an increased risk of GORD. Obese individuals have also been found to be at increased risk. This is mainly due to impairment of the lower oesophageal sphincter as a result of increasing intra-abdominal pressure and subsequent reflux.

Smoking, alcohol and caffeine are also linked to sphincter impairment through enhanced transient sphincter relaxation mechanisms. Consumption of foods with a high fat content may increase an individual's risk due to delayed gastric emptying. From an environmental perspective, studies have demonstrated that *Helicobacter pylori* infection may be protective in reducing the risk of developing GORD.

From a pathophysiological viewpoint, impairment of the lower oesophageal sphincter is deemed to be highly significant in the occurrence of GORD. Normally, the sphincter relaxes during oesophageal peristalsis, and such relaxations are referred to as transient lower oesophageal sphincter relaxations (TLOSRs). However, in individuals with GORD there is an increased frequency of these relaxations. Such relaxations may also occur at an increased frequency in individuals who are known to have a hiatus hernia.

Clinical presentation

The presentation can vary widely, and it is therefore important to keep a broad list of possible differential diagnoses in mind. Patients often present with heartburn and regurgitation. Less frequent symptoms include dysphagia, water brash and a cough (particularly a nocturnal cough).

It is important to specifically ask the patient if they notice symptoms of acid reflux, water brash and retrosternal discomfort when stooping or lying down. They may also find that their symptoms are worse after a large meal or when straining.

Symptoms that should raise concern, and trigger an upper GI endoscopy, include the following:

- odynophagia (this may occur with oesophagitis)
- dysphagia
- protracted vomiting
- weight loss
- anaemia
- age over 55 years or symptoms lasting for > 4 weeks.

Be aware of the patient who was diagnosed with asthma at the age of 50 years and has no typical features of asthma other than a wheeze, and no smoking history to indicate COPD! They often describe a nocturnal cough, no history of atopy, and no benefit from the inhalers they have been given. Some patients may give a history of recurrent chest infections due to the aspiration of gastric contents at night.

Young patients with odynophagia should have a full social and sexual history taken. Bear in mind the possibility of immunosuppression from HIV with underlying candida oesophagitis.

Initial investigations

Much of the investigation of GORD is discussed in the NICE guidelines. The age of the patient and the symptoms that they report will determine which investigations are appropriate. One would investigate a 22-year-old man in a completely different way to a 65-year-old!

- **FBC.** Anaemia should prompt further investigation in any case. However, it may be indicative of a potentially serious underlying diagnosis, such as malignancy. The WCC may be elevated in cases of recurrent aspiration.
- **U&Es.** Although this is uncommon with GORD alone, patients may become dehydrated. Repeated vomiting may result in hypokalaemia.
- **LFTs.** GORD alone is unlikely to cause abnormalities of liver function. Hypoalbuminaemia may result from prolonged malnutrition, but is likely to represent a more serious underlying diagnosis.
- **Clotting screen.** Prior to OGD, clotting factors should be checked to ensure that they are within the normal ranges. An INR of less than 1.5 is preferred prior to endoscopy.
- **ECG.** Any patient who presents with symptoms of chest pain should have an ECG to rule out myocardial ischaemia. Occasionally pains suggestive of GORD are in fact myocardial in origin.
- **CXR.** Look for signs of aspiration pneumonia (usually right base). A large hiatus hernia is not uncommon in the context of GORD. If the patient describes dysphagia, look for possible causes of extrinsic compression from mediastinal masses or a retrosternal goitre.

Further investigations

GORD is classically a clinical diagnosis. An upper GI endoscopy is the gold standard diagnostic investigation to help to confirm the presence of oesophagitis. Other investigations, such as a barium swallow, may be helpful in patients with an oesophageal ring or stricture.

Oesophagogastroduodenoscopy

The grading of oesophagitis is based on the Los Angeles classification:
- LA grade A: mucosal break ≤ 5 mm
- LA grade B: mucosal break > 5mm
- LA grade C: mucosal break continuous between more than two mucosal folds
- LA grade D: mucosal break ≥ 75% of oesophageal circumference.

An upper GI endoscopy also helps to confirm the presence of disease-related complications, such as a stricture or Barrett's oesophagus.

Ambulatory pH monitoring

This is another useful investigation, which involves the introduction of a pH probe trans-nasally to 5 cm above the lower oesophageal sphincter. This allows pH measurements to be recorded over a 24-hour period, with reflux episodes occurring at a pH of < 4. An improvement on this technique is the utilisation of the Bravo capsule, a wireless device that is placed 5–6 cm above the gastro-oesophageal junction. This allows pH measurements to be recorded, typically over a 48-hour period.

Management

The management of GORD involves addressing lifestyle factors, as well as medical and surgical intervention.

Medical management

The mainstay of medical management relies on the use of proton pump inhibitors such as omeprazole or lansoprazole. Other useful but less effective therapies include H_2-receptor antagonists such as ranitidine.

Lifestyle modifications should also be discussed with the patient, and should include the following:
- smoking cessation – offer the option of referral to a smoking cessation clinic
- a reduction in alcohol intake, and avoiding consumption of alcohol just before sleeping
- a reduction in meal size – it is better to eat smaller meals more often
- avoidance of precipitating foods, such as spicy food
- weight reduction in obese patients – it may be helpful to refer the patient to a dietician.

In accordance with NICE guidelines, once evidence of oesophagitis has been confirmed following endoscopy, the patient is commenced on full-dose proton pump inhibitors for up to 2 months. If there is no response to such intervention, a double-dose regimen is utilised for an additional month. If this also proves unsuccessful, the patient is trialled on H_2-receptor antagonists, or a prokinetic agent, for up to 1 month. If symptoms still persist, NICE guidelines recommend that specialist input should be sought, or that double-dose PPI should be used with an H_2-receptor antagonist at bedtime.

Surgical/interventional management

Failure of medical intervention prompts the use of endoscopic and surgical-based therapies. Endoscopic therapies include the use of sutures placed around the lower oesophageal sphincter. Other useful alternatives include the use of radiofrequency waves directed at the sphincter itself to help to reduce the frequency of relaxations. In addition, polymer-based agents such as polyethylene may help to strengthen the sphincter considerably.

With regard to surgical therapies, fundoplication, whereby the fundus is plicated around the lower portion of the oesophagus, has been demonstrated to be a worthwhile form of treatment. Surgical intervention is generally only considered when symptoms are severe and refractory to medical therapies, and pH monitoring has also provided evidence of severe reflux. Fundoplication can be performed either as an open procedure or laparoscopically.

Daily monitoring/investigations

Patients with symptoms of GORD alone are unlikely to be admitted for investigation. However, they may undergo investigation as an inpatient either due to frailty or because there is a suspected serious underlying cause.

1 Observations of vital signs – these are likely to be normal unless there is a separate underlying pathology.
2 Daily examination – this is unlikely to yield anything specific, but is good medical practice.
3 Bloods, including FBC, U&Es and LFTs twice per week if the patient is stable. It is important to perform a clotting screen if the patient is due to go for endoscopy.

Important tips

Endoscopy

Make any requests for endoscopy early on. It is not uncommon for patients who are medically fit for discharge to have to wait in hospital for an endoscopic investigation. Ensure that the form is filled in completely and that it includes a clear explanation of the clinical presentation and the question to be answered.

Previous records

Review the patient's case notes, looking in particular for details of previous investigations of GORD. You will then avoid repeating unnecessary investigations if they have been completed recently.

Future advice

The patient should be advised about lifestyle modifications as discussed above. Any referrals to dieticians and smoking cessation clinics should be made, and the patient should be notified of the date and time of these appointments.

Information to have to hand for ward rounds

1 Up-to-date bloods, including FBC, U&Es and LFTs.
2 An ECG to demonstrate that myocardial ischaemia has been ruled out may be useful.
3 Recent CXR.
4 Results of the most recent endoscopy, or the date when it is booked.
5 Observation chart.

Further reading

- Lundell L, Dent J, Bennett J et al. Endoscopic assessment of esophagitis: clinical and functional correlates and further validation of Los Angeles classification. *Gut* 1999; **45:** 172–80.
- NICE guideline: www.nice.org.uk/nicemedia/pdf/ CG017NICEguideline.pdf

7

Barrett's oesophagus

Epidemiology

Barrett's oesophagus is defined as the metaplastic change of the oesophageal epithelial lining from normal squamous cells to columnar cells. The condition itself is pre-malignant and predisposes to the development of adenocarcinoma, and it commonly develops following long-standing gastro-oesophageal reflux.

Barrett's oesophagus is common in Western populations, and predominantly occurs in individuals aged between 40 and 60 years. Its prevalence reflects the increased occurrence of GORD in this population group.

Aetiology

Risk factors for the development of Barrett's oesophagus include increasing age, Caucasian origin, history of long-standing reflux, obesity, cigarette smoking and alcohol misuse. Studies have demonstrated that *Helicobacter pylori* infection may be protective against the development of Barrett's oesophagus. This may be due to the bacterial production of ammonia or destruction of parietal cells, the end result being a reduction in acid volumes, subsequent reflux and inflammation.

From a genetic perspective, studies have shown that the *CDX2* gene may be implicated, with over-expression resulting in metaplastic changes within the oesophagus.

Clinical presentation

Patients typically present with symptoms allied to gastro-oesophageal reflux, namely heartburn and regurgitation, as well as dysphagia in some cases. Barrett's oesophagus is commonly an incidental endoscopic finding in patients who are undergoing endoscopy for another reason.

Initial investigations

The investigation process usually takes place in the outpatient setting. Initial investigations are likely to be limited, as endoscopy is the diagnostic investigation of choice. Malignancy should always be excluded in patients with so-called 'red flag symptoms', which include the following:

- weight loss
- anaemia
- age over 55 years
- protracted vomiting
- dysphagia and/or odynophagia.

The following initial investigations should be undertaken:

- **FBC.** Microcytic anaemia may indicate an underlying malignancy, or bleeding from another cause. A normocytic anaemia of chronic disease may also be present.
- **U&Es.** Raised serum creatinine and urea levels may occur in the context of dysphagia and odynophagia as a result of dehydration due to reduced oral intake.
- **CXR.** Look closely for a hiatus hernia with a fluid level behind the heart. A CXR is also helpful to look for evidence of recurrent aspiration pneumonias due to GORD, as well as for excluding other causes of retrosternal/chest pain.
- **ECG.** This is a cheap straightforward investigation that may help to exclude atypical presentations of myocardial infarction.
- **Clotting screen.** If the patient is going for an endoscopic procedure, check the clotting factors and ensure that they are within normal ranges.

Further investigations

Oesophagogastroduodenoscopy

An upper GI endoscopy is the gold standard initial investigation. The Prague C and M criteria is often used to assess the circumferential (C) and maximum (M) extent of the Barrett's oesophagus segment. Biopsies enable histological assessment of the epithelium and the detection of goblet cells which are characteristic of the condition (see section on diagnostic criteria below).

Capsule endoscopy

Capsule endoscopy has also been utilised with much success in the detection of Barrett's oesophagus. This investigation is often only available in a tertiary centre for gastroenterology. It involves the patient swallowing a small 'capsule' which contains a camera and light source. This transmits images to a data recorder, and the recorded images can then be reviewed at a later date.

Newer imaging techniques include combining the use of autofluorescence and endoscopy, which utilises blue light to detect fluorescence within the epithelium. Neoplastic tissue appears blue-violet in colour, which is useful in the detection of adenocarcinoma formation arising from Barrett's oesophagus.

In accordance with the British Society of Gastroenterology (BSG) guidelines, individuals with no evidence of dysplastic changes should have a follow-up endoscopy every 2 years. Individuals with evidence of low-grade dysplasia should ideally be followed up every 6 months. Biopsy samples are quadrant in nature, and are taken every 2 cm within the columnar segment.

Diagnostic criteria

The diagnosis of Barrett's oesophagus is based on the following criteria:
1 salmon-pink-coloured tongues of epithelium that project upwards into the oesophagus
2 the presence of goblet cells on histological examination of the oesophageal epithelium.

However, criterion 2 is not universal, and a diagnosis of the condition can be made solely on the basis of the occurrence of criterion 1.

Management

Medical management

To date, there is no evidence to suggest that either H_2-receptor blockers or proton pump inhibitors have any effect on reversal of metaplastic change. However, it should be recognised that both H_2-receptor blockers and proton pump inhibitors do have a role in patients with GORD and erosive oesophagitis.

Studies have demonstrated the potential use of NSAIDs in reducing the risk of Barrett's oesophagus and carcinoma formation. However, this is not currently recommended as a form of treatment.

The mainstay of management is the use of high-dose proton pump inhibitors coupled with endoscopic mucosal resection or ablative therapies involving argon plasma coagulation, cryotherapy with liquid nitrogen, or delivery of radiofrequency waves. Patients with low-grade dysplastic change should be followed up with repeat endoscopy at 6 months. Those with high-grade dysplasia require follow-up endoscopy at 3 months, unless there is also mucosal irregularity, in which case endoscopic mucosal resection is recommended. Patients with high-grade dysplasia should be discussed with the surgeons in an MDT meeting to decide about the possibility of oesophagectomy.

Surgical management

For patients with high-grade dysplastic changes, surgical intervention in the form of an oesophagectomy is key. For those who are not fit to undergo surgery, ablative or mucosal resection techniques are beneficial.

It has also been debated whether anti-reflux therapies may be useful, as in the case of GORD. However, such interventions are not currently recommended for the treatment of Barrett's oesophagus.

Further reading

- Liu T, Zhang X, So CK *et al*. Regulation of CDX2 expression by promoter methylation, and effects of CDX2 transfection on morphology and gene expression of human esophageal epithelial cells. *Carcinogenesis* 2007; **28:** 488–96.
- Sharma P, Dent J, Armstrong D *et al*. The development and validation of an endoscopic grading system for Barrett's esophagus: the Prague C & M criteria. *Gastroenterology* 2006; **131:** 1392–9.
- Playford RJ. New British Society of Gastroenterology (BSG) guidelines for the diagnosis and management of Barrett's oesophagus. *Gut* 2006; **55:** 442.

8

Oesophageal cancer

Oesophageal cancers are commonly squamous-cell carcinomas or adeno-carcinomas. Squamous-cell carcinomas are typically located in the upper or middle third of the oesophagus, whereas adenocarcinomas are located in the lower third.

Epidemiology

Oesophageal cancer is particularly common in Northern Iran, China and southern Russia. In the UK in 2007 there were roughly 8000 cases of oesophageal cancer diagnosed, with a male to female ratio of almost 2:1 according to Cancer Research UK.[1]

Aetiology

Cigarette smoking is associated with the development of squamous-cell carcinomas and adenocarcinomas. Dietary factors are also important, and there is an increased risk of development of these carcinomas in individuals with a diet low in fruit and vegetables and high in salt-containing foods.

Squamous-cell carcinomas are specifically associated with alcohol misuse, achalasia, tylosis and Plummer–Vinson syndrome. Adenocarcinomas are commonly linked to the occurrence of Barrett's oesophagus, which develops following long-standing gastro-oesophageal reflux disease.

With regards to genetic abnormalities, studies have shown an increasing association with p53, p27, E-cadherin and α- and β-catenin-based mutations.

Clinical presentation

Common symptoms include dysphagia, odynophagia and weight loss. The history of onset of dysphagia is important. Patients often initially experience dysphagia to solids, which subsequently progresses to liquids as well. The experience of food 'sticking' may also occur. However, the level bears no relevance to the site of the tumour.

Individuals may also suffer from a cough, hoarse voice, retrosternal pain or discomfort, and dyspnoea. Examination findings may reveal evidence of hepatomegaly and supraclavicular lymphadenopathy. However, system examination may also be completely normal.

Initial investigations

- **FBC.** The most common finding is a microcytic anaemia. This is often an iron-deficiency anaemia secondary to bleeding. The platelet count may be elevated. The WCC may be elevated in cases of aspiration pneumonia.
- **Anaemia screen.** Tests should include iron studies, vitamin B_{12}, folic acid and thyroid function (and haemoglobinopathy screen in selected patients). Ensure that the anaemia screen is done before transfusion of blood products!
- **U&Es.** Patients with dysphagia or odynophagia may be dehydrated and suffering from pre-renal failure.
- **LFTs.** Metastatic spread may occur, resulting in deranged liver function. Hypoalbuminaemia may occur in more advanced stages of disease, as a result of malnutrition combined with the catabolic state of malignancy.
- **Clotting screen.** A baseline clotting screen should be performed if the patient is to undergo an OGD.
- **Group and save.** A routine sample should be sent, as the patient may require transfusion.
- **CXR.** Look for evidence of metastatic spread and aspiration pneumonia.

Further investigations

Barium swallow

Historically, the initial diagnostic investigation is a barium swallow. This can help to graphically differentiate between the different underlying pathological processes that can result in dysphagia, such as malignancy and achalasia. However, in clinical practice, patients often undergo an OGD as the initial investigation, as they may be anaemic and have a history of dysphagia. Discuss further investigations with a gastroenterology specialist registrar or consultant.

Oesophagogastroduodenoscopy

OGD is a useful diagnostic tool, as it allows visualisation of the oesophageal mucosa. Images can be stored and biopsies taken. Multiple biopsies should be taken at any one time.

CT staging

If malignancy is confirmed, a staging CT should be undertaken. This involves imaging of the chest, abdomen and pelvis. Staging of the disease will influence the potential management options and indicate whether curative resection may be possible.

Management

Medical management

The management of oesophageal cancer is dependent on the extent of disease spread. Advanced disease is treated with chemotherapy-based agents such as fluorouracil and irinotecan.

Radiotherapy is often considered for patients with squamous-cell carcinoma who are generally not fit to undergo surgery.

Photodynamic therapy in conjunction with proton pump inhibitor use has been shown to be beneficial in the eradication of superficial oesophageal cancer.

Surgical management

Localised disease is treated surgically using either a trans-thoracic or a trans-hiatal approach. The trans-thoracic approach is typically right-sided, resulting in the formation of an oesophago-gastric anastomosis in the upper chest (Ivor Lewis technique) or in the neck. The trans-hiatal approach involves the formation of an anastomosis in the neck, and is associated with fewer operative complications overall. This is high-risk surgery with a significant mortality rate, which may be as high as 10%.

Palliative management

For patients with incurable disease, symptom control, namely of dysphagia, is essential. This is often achieved through radiotherapy or cisplatin-based chemotherapy. Alternatively, patients may benefit from balloon insertion and dilatation or stent placement. Complications of stent placement include migration and subsequent gastro-oesophageal reflux.

Daily monitoring/investigations

1 Close observation of vital signs.
2 Daily examination, looking specifically for signs of dehydration, and initiating IV fluids as necessary.
3 Twice weekly bloods, including FBC, U&Es, CRP and LFTs.

Information to have to hand for ward rounds

1 Up-to-date bloods, including FBC, U&Es, LFTs and CRP.
2 Results of barium swallow/OGD, or the date when it is booked.
3 Results of any histology.
4 Observation chart for temperature and haemodynamic status.

Reference

1 www.cancerresearchuk.org

Further reading

- Nakanishi Y, Ochiai A, Akimoto S *et al.* Expression of E-cadherin, alpha-catenin, beta-catenin and plakoglobin in esophageal carcinomas and its prognostic significance: immunohistochemical analysis of 96 lesions. *Oncology* 1997; **54:** 158–65.

9

Gastric cancer

Epidemiology

Gastric cancer is the fourth most common cancer worldwide. The male to female ratio is 2:1. The incidence of gastric cancer is highest in certain parts of Asia, such as Japan and China, as well as in some parts of South America. The lowest incidence is in North America.

Aetiology

The development of gastric cancer has been shown to be associated with increased consumption of foods with a high salt content, and a low intake of fruit and vegetables. *Helicobacter pylori* infection and cigarette smoking have also been shown to be associated with gastric cancer.

Genetic mutations of the E-cadherin gene have been shown to increase the risk of gastric cancer, as has the STK11 mutation seen in Peutz–Jeghers syndrome. Genetic alterations within inflammatory mediator genes are also common, including interleukin 1β and interferon-γ receptor 1. In the vast majority of cases, gastric cancers develop sporadically as a result of chromosomal abnormalities.

Clinical presentation

Patients with early-stage disease may present with weight loss, abdominal pain and nausea. Appetite may be poor, and patients often give a history of early satiety at mealtimes. In the later stages of disease, dysphagia, a palpable abdominal mass or ascites may occur. Protracted vomiting can also occur if there is gastric outlet obstruction by the tumour.

Clinical examination may reveal nothing at all in many cases. Important clinical findings include cachexia, pallor of anaemia, and lymphadenopathy (specifically looking for Virchow's node in the left supraclavicular fossa).

Initial investigations

- **FBC.** There may be normocytic anaemia of chronic disease or, more commonly, a microcytic anaemia as a result of bleeding from the tumour. There may also be an elevated platelet count.
- **U&Es.** Raised urea and creatinine levels may be a result of dehydration due to either reduced oral intake or vomiting. In the later stages, malnutrition can result in low urea and creatinine levels, due to reduced muscle mass. Electrolyte disturbance (hypokalaemia and hypochloraemia) may result from vomiting, and there should be appropriate supplementation.
- **LFTs.** Metastatic spread may result in derangement of liver function, necessitating further investigation. Hypoalbuminaemia is likely to occur in the later stages of disease, due to the combined effects of malnutrition and the catabolic state of malignancy.
- **Bone profile.** Hypercalcaemia may be the result of either dehydration or metastatic spread to the bones.
- **Clotting screen.** If there is metastatic spread to the liver, synthetic function may be impaired, resulting in a prolonged PT/INR. This should be corrected appropriately, usually by administering vitamin K.
- **AXR.** An abdominal film should be requested in patients who present with obstruction. Look for evidence of Rigler's sign (air on both sides of the bowel wall).
- **Erect CXR.** Features of perforation may be detected by air under the diaphragm. A large gastric bubble with a fluid level may be seen in gastric outflow obstruction.

Further investigations

Oesophagogastroduodenoscopy

This is an important investigation, as it reveals a diagnosis in approximately 95% of cases, and allows biopsies to be taken for a histological diagnosis. Other conditions, such as peptic ulcer disease, which may present with similar features, can also be investigated at the same time.

Barium meal

A barium meal can help to diagnose cases of suspected gastric outflow obstruction. This is particularly useful in cases where the gastric tumour prevents the physical passage of the scope, and it can help to provide a crude estimate of the extent of tumour bulk.

Endoscopic ultrasound

This investigation is often only available at centres with a tertiary gastroenterology service. EUS can be used to help to identify the depth of penetration of tumour, as well as the extent of invasion into surrounding structures, and to obtain biopsy specimens for a histological diagnosis. It is therefore an extremely useful tool in the planning of treatment.

CT

Staging CT imaging is required to help to decide on the appropriate management, and to determine whether curative surgical resection is likely to be possible. CT imaging of the chest, abdomen and pelvis is required. If contrast is to be used, the patient may require pre-hydration with IV fluids.

PET scan

If curative surgical resection is to be considered, a PET scan is important to accurately ascertain whether there is any lymph node involvement.

Tumour markers

CEA and CA19-9 do not have a role in diagnosis, but can be used after the initiation of treatment to assess its effectiveness, and also as surveillance for disease recurrence. However, these tumour markers are not present in all patients. CEA is present in around 50% of patients with gastric cancer, and CA19-9 is present in only around 20% of them.

Management
Medical management
Diet

Malnutrition is a significant problem as a result of both reduced appetite and the catabolic state of malignancy. Dietary requirements should be ascertained by a dietician and supplemented as appropriate. It is important to optimise the patient's condition prior to either chemotherapy or surgery.

Chemotherapy

A platinum-based regimen is commonly utilised, and can be used either in the neoadjuvant setting to reduce tumour bulk prior to surgery, or in the adjuvant setting of post-operative recurrence. Chemotherapeutic regimens are complex, and a discussion of them is beyond the scope of this book.

Radiotherapy

Although pre-, intra- and post-operative radiotherapy is used, this remains controversial. Radiotherapy has beneficial effects with regard to pain relief and relief of obstruction, and is commonly used in the palliative setting for these purposes.

Novel therapies

The pathogenesis of gastric cancer involves an array of growth factors, and studies have demonstrated the potential role of inhibitors targeted against epidermal and vascular endothelial growth factor receptors.

Surgical management

Surgical management is directed at those gastric cancers which are localised to the mucosa or sub-mucosa with no evidence of distant metastases or lymph node involvement. This is referred to as curative resection. Surgery may also be used in the palliative setting in some cases.

Important tips

Multidisciplinary management

Gastric cancer is complex and requires a multidisciplinary approach to care. The team is likely to consist of gastroenterologists, upper GI surgeons, oncologists, specialist nurses and dieticians. In some cases, involvement of the palliative care team may be required. It is important that this team is assembled at an early stage of the admission.

Information to have to hand for ward rounds

1 Up-to-date bloods, including FBC, U&Es, LFTs, CRP and tumour markers.
2 The results of any imaging.
3 Endoscopy reports.
4 Histology results.
5 Observation chart for temperature and haemodynamic status.

Further reading

- Guilford PJ, Hopkins JB, Grady WM *et al.* E-cadherin germline mutations define an inherited cancer syndrome dominated by diffuse gastric cancer. *Human Mutation* 1999; **14:** 249–55.
- Shinmura K, Goto M, Tao H *et al.* A novel STK11 germline mutation

in two siblings with Peutz–Jeghers syndrome complicated by primary gastric cancer. *Clinical Genetics* 2005; **67:** 81–6.

- Canedo P, Corso G, Pereira F *et al.* The interferon gamma receptor 1 (*IFNGR1*) –56C/T gene polymorphism is associated with increased risk of early gastric carcinoma. *Gut* 2008; **57:** 1504–8.
- El-Omar EM, Carrington M, Chow WH *et al.* Interleukin-1 polymorphisms associated with increased risk of gastric cancer. *Nature* 2000; **404:** 398–402.
- Gastrointestinal Tumor Study Group. The concept of locally advanced gastric cancer: effect of treatment on outcome. *Cancer* 1990; **66:** 2324–30.
- Cunningham D, Allum WH, Stenning SP *et al.* Perioperative chemotherapy versus surgery alone for resectable gastroesophageal cancer. *New England Journal of Medicine* 2006; **355:** 11–20.
- Ohtsu A. Chemotherapy for metastatic gastric cancer: past, present, and future. *Journal of Gastroenterology* 2008; **43:** 256–64.

10

Inflammatory bowel disease

Epidemiology/aetiology

Ulcerative colitis (UC) and Crohn's disease (CD) are inflammatory diseases of the gastrointestinal mucosa. They are complex disorders which present in a variety of ways, often run a relapsing and remitting course, and may cause chronic ill health.

In UC, mucosal inflammation is limited to the colon, whereas in CD any segment of the GI tract from the mouth to the anus may be involved. It is usually possible to distinguish between UC and CD on the basis of clinical, radiological, endoscopic and pathology investigations. However, in approximately 5–15% of patients this is not possible, and in these cases the patient's condition is known as indeterminate colitis.

UC and CD affect approximately 1 in every 400 members of the population, with 6000–12 000 new cases of UC and 3000–6000 new cases of CD diagnosed annually in the UK. The number of people diagnosed with CD is rising particularly rapidly.

Three major classes of drugs are used to treat inflammatory bowel disease, namely steroids, immunomodulators and biological agents. Steroids are used to induce remission in acute flares, and immunomodulators (azathioprine, methotrexate and mercaptopurine) are used to maintain remissions and modify the disease pattern. CD may also respond to the use of antibiotics and liquid diets (elemental and polymeric). In both diseases surgery may be helpful for removing strictures or damaged areas of bowel, while colectomy may be curative for patients with UC. New biological agents such as infliximab are increasingly changing the management of inflammatory bowel disease.

Ulcerative colitis

The incidence of UC is approximately 10–20 per 100 000 people per year (approximately 1 in every 500 people in the UK), with a peak incidence in the 10–40 years age group. There is no gender difference in incidence, but there is a marked difference in racial incidence, with Ashkenazi Jews having a particularly high burden of disease.

UC is typically characterised in terms of the extent of the disease. Distal disease is confined to the rectum (proctitis) or to the rectum and sigmoid colon (proctosigmoiditis). More extensive disease includes left-sided colitis (to the splenic flexure), extensive colitis (to the hepatic flexure) and pancolitis (affecting the whole colon).

The cause of inflammatory bowel disease remains unknown, but it appears to involve dysregulation of the GI mucosal immune response to environmental triggers in genetically susceptible individuals, with a loss of tolerance of the indigenous enteric flora or that found in the bloodstream.

Around 15% of UC patients have a positive family history of the disease, and genetic susceptibility has been linked to chromosomes 12 and 16. Genetic susceptibility is less strong in UC than in CD, and the pattern of disease may be more related to HLA genotype. For example, HLA-DR1 is 5 to 11 times more common in patients who require colectomy than in those who do not. Serum and mucosal autoantibodies against intestinal epithelial cells have been identified, and patients may be perinuclear anti-neutrophil cytoplasmic antibodies (pANCA) positive.

UC is more common in non-smokers than in smokers, and is one of the few conditions where smoking appears to offer some protective benefit.

Crohn's disease

This condition is characterised by transmural granulomatous inflammation of any part of the GI tract. It may be defined by location (terminal ileal, colonic, ileocolonic or upper GI) or by pattern of disease (inflammatory, fistulating or stricturing).

The incidence of disease is approximately 70–100 per 100 000 people (1 in every 1000 people in the UK). The peak age of onset is 10–40 years, and the incidence varies little with race, sex or social class. The genetic predisposition in CD is stronger than that in UC. Genes that predispose to up to 40% of small bowel CD have been identified on chromosome 16 (NOD2/CARD16). Other recognised genes in CD are OCTN1 and OCTN2 on chromosome 5 (which may be associated with perianal disease), and DLG5 on chromosome 10.

Smoking is positively associated with CD, which is twice as common in smokers as in non-smokers. Smoking cessation is part of the treatment, as this reduces the risk of relapse, the need for immunosuppression, and the need for surgery.

Clinical presentation

Clinical presentation in inflammatory bowel disease depends on which area of the intestinal tract is inflamed. It is not usually possible to distinguish UC from CD on the basis of symptoms alone, although there may be some indications. CD typically causes more long-term disability than UC, with only 75% of patients fully capable of returning to work a year after diagnosis, and up to 15% of patients unable to work after having the disease for 5–10 years.

TABLE 10.1 Presentation in ulcerative colitis (UC) and Crohn's disease (CD)

ULCERATIVE COLITIS	CROHN'S DISEASE
Gradual-onset diarrhoea with blood and mucus	Abdominal pain
Bowel frequency related to disease severity	Diarrhoea
Crampy abdominal pain	Weight loss
Systemic features during an acute attack (e.g. fever, malaise)	Systemic features more common in CD than in UC
Urgency and tenesmus, particularly if there is rectal disease	Risk of intestinal obstruction, strictures, fistulae or abscesses

TABLE 10.2 Differentiation of ulcerative colitis from Crohn's disease

	ULCERATIVE COLITIS	CROHN'S DISEASE
Clinical		
Bloody diarrhoea	90–100%	50%
Abdominal pain	Very rare	Common
Perianal disease	Very uncommon	30–50%
Sigmoidoscopy		
Rectal sparing	Never	50%
Histology		
Distribution	Mucosal	Transmural
Cellular infiltrate	Polymorphs	Lymphocytes
Goblet-cell depletion	Distorted	Normal
Radiology		
Distribution	Continuous	Discontinuous

(*continued*)

	ULCERATIVE COLITIS	CROHN'S DISEASE
Symmetry	Symmetrical	Asymmetrical
Mucosa	Shallow ulcers	Deep ulcers
Strictures	Very rare	Common
Fistulae	Never	Common

Reprinted from Travis *et al.*[1]

Extra-intestinal manifestations may also occur in 10–20% of patients. These may include the following:
- clubbing
- aphthous ulceration
- erythema nodosum
- pyoderma gangrenosum
- conjunctivitis
- episcleritis
- iritis
- arthritis
- ankylosing spondylitis
- sacroiliitis.

A focused history is of benefit. Particular attention should be paid to the following areas of the history:
- mode of onset of symptoms
- frequency and nature of stool (e.g. watery, bloody, mucus, pus)
- triggers – new foods (e.g. takeaways, meals out)
- family history
- other symptoms (e.g. abdominal pain, fever, malaise, rash, vomiting, mouth ulcers, uveitis)
- travel abroad
- recent hospitalisation
- recent medication (e.g. antacids, antibiotics)
- any other medical problems.

Initial investigations
- **FBC.** Anaemia is common in severe attacks or chronic disease (normocytic). Thrombocythaemia may indicate active inflammation.
- **U&Es.** Hypokalaemia, hypophosphataemia and hypomagnesaemia are more common in diarrhoea.
- **LFTs.** Albumin levels may be low in chronic inflammatory bowel disease, and this is a prognostic marker. Primary sclerosing cholangitis

is particularly associated with UC, and to a lesser extent with CD. ALP is initially elevated, followed by bilirubin. If primary sclerosing cholangitis is suspected, send ANA and anti-smooth muscle antibodies (SMA).

- **ESR and CRP.** These indicate the level of underlying inflammation.
- **Blood cultures.** Must be sent if the patient is febrile.
- **Stool samples.** Send samples for microscopy, culture, ova, cysts and parasite screen, and *Clostridium difficile*. It is important to exclude infection as an exacerbating factor.
- **CXR and AXR.** Look for evidence of perforation and radiological evidence of disease activity (e.g. toxic dilatation, loss of haustral folds, etc.).

Further investigations

Colonoscopy/flexible sigmoidoscopy

In the acutely colitic patient, flexible sigmoidoscopy may be of benefit. This will help to provide information about disease activity. Colonoscopy will usually form the mainstay of investigation of inflammatory bowel disease, allowing both biopsies and images of the bowel to be taken.

Bowel preparation is extremely important for optimising the quality of the images that are obtained. You must consult your local hospital guidelines to confirm the preferred bowel preparation, and ensure that this is given at the right time before the procedure.

Patients who are sent for endoscopic procedures must have IV access. They must provide written consent for both flexible sigmoidoscopy and colonoscopy. You will not be required to do this, as junior doctors (house officers and senior house officers) are not competent to perform these investigations.

Oesophagogastroduodenoscopy

This may be a useful adjunct in a patient with CD affecting the upper GI tract, allowing both biopsies and images to be taken during the investigation. The patient must be nil by mouth for at least 6 hours before their OGD. Consent must be obtained by someone who is competent to perform the investigation. The patient will require IV access.

CT abdomen

In the acutely unwell patient, a CT may be helpful for identifying fistulas, collections and abscesses, and for planning pre-surgery.

Small bowel imaging

In the instance of Crohn's disease, it is important to consider imaging modalities to look at the small bowel. Barium follow-through studies are readily available in the majority of trusts, however MRI is usually less accessible. Quantifying the extent of disease is extremely important with regard to management and prognosis.

Assessing the severity of IBD

- General examination – assess the patient's hydration status and the severity of the attack (tachycardia, abdominal distension and evidence of bowel perforation).
- Assess disease severity with the Truelove and Witt score for UC (*see* Table 10.3), and with the Crohn's Disease Activity Index (CDAI) for CD (*see* Table 10.4).
- Assess the patient for extra-intestinal manifestations (e.g. oral ulceration, rashes, uveitis).
- Always perform a digital rectal examination. Look in particular for evidence of peri-anal skin changes (e.g. skin tags, ulcers, fissures).
- Your senior may consider whether a sigmoidoscopy or colonoscopy is required.

TABLE 10.3 Truelove and Witt score

FEATURES	MILD	MODERATE	SEVERE
Number of motions/day	< 4	4–6	> 6
PR bleeding	Small	Moderate	Large
Temperature (°C)	Afebrile	37.1–37.8	> 37.8
Pulse rate (beats/minute)	< 70	70–90	> 90
Hb (g/dl)	> 11	10.5–11.0	< 10.5
ESR (mm/hour)	< 20	20–30	> 30

PR, per rectum; Hb, haemoglobin; ESR, erythrocyte sedimentation rate.

When calculating the CDAI, one point is added for each of the following sets of complications:
- arthralgia or arthritis
- iritis or uveitis
- erythema nodosum, pyoderma gangrenosum or aphthous ulcers
- anal fissures, fistulae or abscesses
- other bowel-related fistulae
- fever (> 37.4 °C) during the previous 7 days.

Severe CD is defined as a CDAI score of > 450.

TABLE 10.4 Crohn's Disease Activity Index (CDAI)

VARIABLE	WEIGHTING FACTOR
Number of liquid or soft stools each day for 7 days	× 2
Abdominal pain (0 = least severe, 3 = most severe) each day for 7 days	× 5
General well-being (0 = best, 4 = worst) each day for 7 days	× 7
Taking Lomotil or opiates for diarrhoea	× 30
Presence of an abdominal mass (0 = none, 2 = questionable, 5 = definite)	× 10
Absolute deviation of haematocrit from 47% in men and 42% in women	× 6
Percentage deviation from standard weight	× 1
Presence of complications	× 20

Management

Medical management

When managing an acute flare of inflammatory bowel disease it is important to recognise which patients will require admission to hospital for treatment (patients with moderate to severe features as assessed by the Truelove and Witt score and the CDAI score) and, of these, which will require surgery for symptoms that fail to settle.

Other possible causes of the patient's presentation on this occasion must be excluded (e.g. gastrointestinal infection, bacterial overgrowth, fibrotic strictures, dysmotility, gallstones and bile salt malabsorption).

Steroids (typically hydrocortisone) to control mucosal inflammation are the mainstay of treatment in acute inflammatory bowel disease. These are usually given intravenously (e.g. 50–100 mg hydrocortisone four times a day). Other drugs, such as 5-aminosalicylic acid (ASA) agents, are used to maintain remission. These are often stopped in the acute setting, as they may worsen symptoms.

Other options for both acute management and remission management are cyclosporine and infliximab, discussion of which is beyond the remit of this book.

- Care should be shared between gastroenterologists and general/colorectal surgeons.
- Early involvement of IBD specialist nurses is important.
- IV steroids are the mainstay of treatment (e.g. hydrocortisone 100 mg four times a day).

- Rectal steroids should be given as tolerated (e.g. predfoam enemas, one twice a day).
- ASA agents are poorly tolerated in unwell patients, and should be stopped.
- Give IV fluids and potassium supplementation (maintain potassium levels at > 4.5 mmol/l, as this reduces the risk of colonic dilatation).
- Consider blood transfusion if Hb is < 7 g/dl, or < 10 g/dl in very unwell or elderly patients, or in the presence of multiple comorbidities.
- Give DVT prophylaxis (e.g. low-molecular-weight heparin, such as enoxaparin 40 mg subcutaneously once a day), as patients with acute colitis are pro-coagulant.
- It is important to maintain nutrition. Patients should be nil by mouth if obstruction, dilatation or perforation is suspected. Nutritional supplements may be indicated, and the involvement of a dietician is strongly recommended. The patient's weight and serum albumin level should be monitored. In Crohn's disease, liquid diets (elemental diets) may have a role in treatment.
- Multiple stool samples are required to exclude infection (MC&S, *Clostridium difficile*, ova, cysts and parasites) are required. Liaise with the microbiology lab if the patient has recently travelled abroad.
- An AXR should be taken on the day of admission, and this must be repeated urgently if the patient deteriorates. Inspect in particular for evidence of free air (which may indicate a perforation of the bowel), dilatation of the bowel (to a diameter of > 5.5 cm in the colon or > 9 cm in the caecum) and differential air/fluid levels (which suggest obstruction).

Surgical management

Patients must be assessed formally on day 3 in order to identify those who are not responsive to medical therapy. These patients require referral for surgical review. Around 40% of patients will be in remission by day 3, and 30% will have deteriorated and will require surgery. Indications for surgery include the following:

- severe haemorrhage
- toxic megacolon
- perforation (free or walled-off)
- if after day 3 stool frequency is > 8 stools/day, or stool frequency is 3–8 stools/day with a CRP of > 45 mg/l, there is an 85% probability that colectomy will be needed.

Daily monitoring/investigations

1 Close observation of vital signs. Observations four times a day are routine. However, they may need to be more frequent if the patient is unwell.
2 Daily review of clinical condition, stool charts, food charts and the patient's weight.
3 Daily examination, looking specifically for evidence of bleeding, hydration and nutrition status, and evidence of sepsis, obstruction and perforation.
4 Daily bloods, including FBC, U&Es and LFTs (specifically albumin, which has prognostic value). CRP and ESR should be measured on alternate days, and blood cultures should be taken if the patient has a temperature.

Important tips

Documentation

The Truelove and Witt score or CDAI score should be calculated on admission. This will provide an indication of the severity of the flare. It also provides a means of monitoring improvement or deterioration over time. These scores will help to decide whether the patient can be managed as an inpatient or outpatient, what treatment is appropriate, and whether surgery is indicated.

Microbiology

A minimum of three stool cultures should be sent for MC&S. In some cases it may also be appropriate to send stool samples for ova, cysts and parasites. Cytomegalovirus (CMV) should be considered in patients who are on immunosuppressant treatment. CMV detection involves sending a bowel biopsy specimen and PCR for CMV.

Stool chart

An accurate stool chart must be kept. It is often easiest to ask the patient to fill this out him- or herself. Ensure that the frequency, stool type, colour, consistency, and presence of pus, mucus and/or blood are all documented clearly.

Thromboprophylaxis

Any patient admitted to hospital who is not mobile must have thromboprophylaxis considered. Patients with inflammatory bowel disease are at particular risk of thromboembolism in an acute flare, as they are in a pro-coagulant state. Bloody stool is not a contraindication to giving thromboprophylaxis.

Joint care

Patients with inflammatory bowel disease should be managed jointly under the care of surgeons and gastroenterologists. Both specialties should be involved from an early stage in the admission.

Thiopurinemethyltransferase (TPMT) levels

Early in the admission, check the patient's serum TPMT levels. TPMT is an enzyme that deactivates 6-mercaptopurine. Genetic polymorphisms of TPMT can lead to an accumulation of azathioprine and result in toxicity. Patients with UC should have their fasting plasma cholesterol and magnesium levels checked, in the event that cyclosporine treatment may be needed. Both hypocholesterolaemia (serum cholesterol < 120 mg/dl) and hypomagnesaemia (serum magnesium < 1.5 mg/dl) significantly increase the risk of seizures in patients who have been treated with intravenous cyclosporine.

Electrolytes

Ensure that serum potassium levels are always kept above 4.5 mmol/l, as this has been shown to reduce the risk of toxic dilatation.

Discharge care

Before discharge, ensure that the patient has the following information:
- details of follow-up clinic appointment
- written information about steroid-tapering regimens, the side-effects of their medication, and the warning signs of a disease flare
- the contact details of an IBD specialist nurse who can give them advice and also expedite appointments in an emergency
- the contact details of relevant patient support groups.
  In addition:
- assess the patient's need for bone and GI protection if long-term steroid therapy is required
- ensure that the GP has a clear, up-to-date and legible copy of the patient's investigations and treatment plan. This may circumvent many problems in the long term
- provide the patient with smoking cessation advice and support.

Information to have to hand for ward rounds

1 Up-to-date bloods, including FBC, U&Es, CRP and LFTs.
2 Observation chart.
3 Stool chart – ensure that the frequency and consistency of motions, and the presence of blood, is noted.
4 The results of stool cultures.

5 The results of the most recent AXR.
6 The results of any recent imaging (colonoscopy, barium studies, CT and MRI scans) and biopsies.

Reference

1 Travis S, Ahmad T, Collier J *et al*. *Pocket Consultant Gastroenterology*, 3rd edn. Oxford: Wiley-Blackwell; 2005.

Further reading

- National Association for Colitis and Crohn's Disease (NACC): www.nacc.org.uk
- Sartor R and Sandborn W, eds. *Kirsner's Inflammatory Bowel Diseases*, 6th edn. New York: Saunders; 2004.
- Travis S, Ahmad T, Collier J *et al*. *Pocket Consultant Gastroenterology*, 3rd edn. Oxford: Wiley-Blackwell; 2005.
- Truelove SC and Witts LJ. Cortisone in ulcerative colitis: final report on a therapeutic trial. *British Medical Journal* 1955; **2:** 1041–8.
- Best WR, Becktel JM, Singleton JW *et al*. Development of a Crohn's disease activity index. National Cooperative Crohn's Disease Study. *Gastroenterology* 1976; **70:** 439–44.
- De Groen PC, Aksamit AJ, Rakela J *et al*. Central nervous system toxicity after liver transplantation. The role of cyclosporine and cholesterol. *New England Journal of Medicine* 1987; **317:** 861–6.
- European Crohn's and Colitis Organisation (ECCO) guidelines. www.ecco-ibd.eu/index.php/publications/ecco-guidelines
- Carter M, Lobo A and Travis S, on behalf of the IBD Section of the British Society of Gastroenterology. Guidelines for the management of inflammatory bowel disease in adults. *Gut* 2004; **53(Suppl. 5):** v1–16.

11

Constipation

Epidemiology
Constipation is commonly seen in the Western population, where it has an estimated incidence of 2–27%. It is more prevalent in women than in men, and may be more common in the non-white population.

Aetiology
Aetiology is dependent on the specific form of constipation in question. There are three main forms, namely functional (normal-transit) constipation, defecatory disorders and slow-transit constipation.

Functional constipation
In this form of constipation, stool transit and frequency are normal. The causes are diverse, and may be neurological, psychological or psychosomatic in origin.

Defecatory disorders
These disorders are commonly due to abnormalities of the anal sphincter or the pelvic floor.

Slow-transit constipation
This form of constipation is commonly seen in young women. Histopathology studies have demonstrated abnormalities in certain neurotransmitters, namely substance P, VIP and nitric oxide, with a reduction in the number of interstitial cells of Cajal (the cells involved in the regulation of GI tract motility).

Clinical presentation

Patients typically present with reduced frequency of bowel motion or the passage of hard stool. Rectal bleeding may occur, and may indicate sinister pathology such as cancer. Pain during defecation could indicate a fissure, or tenesmus from a rectal carcinoma. Patients may also present with overflow diarrhoea secondary to constipation itself.

The patient should be examined for the presence of perianal scars, fissures and external haemorrhoids. Assessment of the perineum during rest and straining is also important, in order to determine pelvic floor muscle function during defecation. All patients must of course be examined per rectum for assessment of anal tone and the presence of masses.

Initial investigations

Constipation is unlikely to result in the admission of a patient, but may result in outpatient investigation. That said, constipation is a frequently encountered problem during hospital stays. It is important to rule out potentially correctable or sinister causes of constipation. A close inspection of the patient's drug chart is required, as constipation is frequently iatrogenic (e.g. secondary to opiate-containing drugs, calcium-channel blockers, anti-depressants and some anti-emetics).

- **Digital rectal examination.** This is imperative in all cases of constipation, and is frequently missed!
- **FBC.** A change in bowel habit and/or constipation may be the result of an underlying gastrointestinal malignancy. A microcytic anaemia or anaemia of chronic disease may be present.
- **TFTs.** Hypothyroidism is associated with constipation, and therefore blood tests would reveal a low T_4 and raised TSH.
- **Serum calcium levels.** Hypercalcaemia can result in constipation. If hypercalcaemia is noted, the patient should be treated and further investigated by measuring PTH, vitamin D and ALP levels.
- **AXR.** An abdominal film should not be requested for constipation alone. However, it may be appropriate in order to exclude obstruction.

Further investigations

Colonoscopy

Colonic malignancy may present with constipation. Colonoscopy allows the bowel lumen to be visualised and biopsies to be obtained for a histological diagnosis.

Colonic transit time
Colonic transit time can be measured by using radio-opaque markers. Retention of more than 20% of markers 120 hours after ingestion indicates prolonged transit.

Manometry
Anorectal manometry is useful for assessment of anal sphincter pressures as well as rectal sensation.

Balloon expulsion
Balloon expulsion involves the introduction of a balloon filled with water or air into the rectum. The patient's ability to expel the balloon is then assessed. If they fail to expel it after a 2-minute period, this is indicative of a defecatory disorder.

Defecography
Defecography involves the introduction of barium per rectum. It allows radiological assessment of defecation and the detection of possible structural abnormalities.

Diagnostic criteria
Constipation encompasses several concepts, including the passage of hard stool, infrequent bowel evacuation, and a sense of incomplete evacuation.

Functional constipation, in which there is no notable structural or biochemical abnormality that can account for the presence of constipation, has been defined by the Rome III diagnostic criteria as including two or more of the following:
1 (a) Straining during at least 25% of defecations.
   (b) Lumpy or hard stools for at least 25% of defecations.
   (c) A sensation of incomplete evacuation for at least 25% of defecations.
   (d) A sensation of anorectal obstruction or blockage for at least 25% of defecations.
   (e) The use of manual manoeuvres to facilitate at least 25% of defecations (e.g. digital evacuation, support of the pelvic floor).
   (f) Fewer than three defecations per week.
2 Loose stools are rarely present without the use of laxatives.
3 Insufficient criteria for irritable bowel syndrome (IBS).

For a label of functional constipation, the above criteria must have been fulfilled for the last 3 months, with symptom onset at least 6 months prior to diagnosis.

Management

Medical management

Initial management of patients with constipation involves increased fluid intake. Fibre is useful for individuals with normal-transit or slow-transit constipation.

Osmotic laxatives such as lactulose or polyethelene glycol are suitable for those who demonstrate a poor response to fibre supplements. However, osmotic laxatives do not produce an immediate response, and should be used with caution in patients with renal failure or cardiac dysfunction, as they may lead to electrolyte disturbance and volume overload.

Stimulant laxatives such as senna are used if patients do not respond to either fibre or osmotic laxative preparations. For patients with faecal impaction, enemas such as phosphate are trialled, as they aid bowel contractility and stool softening.

Prokinetic agents that target the 5-HT$_4$ receptor, such as prucalopride, have been demonstrated to be beneficial in the treatment of constipation secondary to irritable bowel syndrome in female patients.

Biofeedback therapy is utilised to treat constipation resulting from a defecatory disorder. It involves enhancing anal sphincter and pelvic floor muscle function, and studies have demonstrated an overall success rate of 67%.

Trials are also under way to analyse the use of botulinum toxin type A, which is injected into the puborectalis muscle, for individuals with defecatory disorders. However, more research is needed before this type of therapy can be deemed both efficacious and safe.

Surgical management

In cases of refractory slow-transit constipation, colonic resection with ileorectal anastomosis may be used.

Further reading

- Rome diagnostic criteria: www.romecriteria.org/pdfs/launch.pdf
- Pare P, Ferrazzi S, Thompson WG *et al.* An epidemiological survey of constipation in Canada: definitions, rates, demographics, and predictors of health care seeking. *American Journal of Gastroenterology* 2001; **96:** 3130–37.
- Johanson JF, Sonnenberg A and Koch TR. Clinical epidemiology of chronic constipation. *Journal of Clinical Gastroenterology* 1989; **11:** 525–36.
- Tzavella K, Riepl RL, Klauser AG *et al.* Decreased substance P levels in rectal biopsies from patients with slow transit constipation. *European Journal of Gastroenterology and Hepatology* 1996; **8:** 1207–11.

- Cortesini C, Cianchi F, Infantino A *et al.* Nitric oxide synthase and VIP distribution in enteric nervous system in idiopathic chronic constipation. *Digestive Diseases and Sciences* 1995; **40:** 2450–5.
- He CL, Burgart L, Wang L *et al.* Decreased interstitial cell of Cajal volume in patients with slow-transit constipation. *Gastroenterology* 2000; **118:** 14–21.
- Camilleri M, Kerstens R, Rykx A *et al.* A placebo-controlled trial of prucalopride for severe chronic constipation. *New England Journal of Medicine* 2008; **358:** 2344–54.
- Enck P. Biofeedback training in disordered defecation: a critical review. *Digestive Diseases and Sciences* 1993; **38:** 1953–60.
- Ron Y, Avni Y, Lukovetski A *et al.* Botulinum toxin type-A in therapy of patients with anismus. *Diseases of the Colon and Rectum* 2001; **44:** 1821–6.

12

Colorectal cancer

Epidemiology

Colorectal cancer is the third most common cancer worldwide. According to the World Health Organization (WHO), the condition accounts for 492 000 deaths per year. The risk of development of colorectal cancer increases significantly after the age of 40 years, with the peak incidence occurring at 65 years of age.

Aetiology

Colorectal cancer primarily arises sporadically, but can also occur as a result of genetic and environmental factors.

From a hereditary perspective, colorectal cancer can develop in individuals with familial adenomatous polyposis (FAP) and hereditary non-polyposis colorectal cancer (HNPCC). Environmental factors of interest include a diet rich in meat, diabetes, smoking, and excessive alcohol consumption. Colorectal cancer may also occur in individuals with inflammatory bowel disease.

The pathogenesis of colorectal cancer depends on two pathways, namely the gatekeeper pathway, which consists of genes responsible for growth regulation (such as the APC gene which is responsible for FAP), and the caretaker pathway, which is characterised by mutations of genes responsible for stability (such as the mismatch repair genes that are responsible for HNPCC).

Clinical presentation

Patients with suspected colorectal cancer may complain of abdominal pain, altered bowel habit, PR bleeding, weight loss and anorexia. In severe cases, colorectal cancer may lead to obstructive symptoms such as vomiting and reduced bowel motion.

It is not uncommon for patients to be asymptomatic or to present with symptoms of anaemia, which is confirmed on routine blood testing.

Physical examination may be completely normal or may reveal a palpable abdominal mass, hepatomegaly, ascites or rectal bleeding.

Initial investigations

- **FBC.** Microcytic anaemia due to iron deficiency may result from prolonged bleeding from the tumour. Malignancy-induced reactive thrombocytosis may also occur.
- **U&Es.** Baseline renal function should be checked, as the patient is likely to require CT imaging with contrast for staging.
- **LFTs.** Metastatic spread to the liver may result in deranged liver function. Hypoalbuminaemia may result from malnutrition combined with the catabolism of malignancy.
- **Serum calcium.** Metastatic spread to the bones may result in raised serum calcium levels.
- **Iron studies.** These are likely to reveal iron deficiency with a low serum ferritin level, low serum iron levels, and high or normal transferrin saturation.
- **CXR.** Pulmonary metastatic spread may be visible on a plain film CXR. Occasionally patients present acutely with bowel perforation at the site of the tumour, and an erect CXR may be helpful to look for free air under the hemidiaphragm.
- **AXR.** Colorectal cancer occasionally presents with bowel obstruction.

Further investigations

Colonoscopy

This is the gold standard investigation of choice. It allows for diagnosis of the lesion as well as anatomical placement, and enables biopsies to be taken for histological confirmation.

Double-contrast barium enema

Double-contrast barium enema is often used pre-operatively to help to outline the sinister lesion more accurately. With improving technology in CT imaging, contrast studies are less commonly used in this context.

CT pneumocolon

This is a less invasive investigative technique than colonoscopy, and allows a 'virtual colonoscopy' to be performed. It is particularly useful in patients who are frail and who may not tolerate a colonoscopy.

CT scan

Imaging of the chest, abdomen and pelvis is required for staging of the malignancy. This has ramifications with regards to the management that is appropriate for the patient, and also whether curative surgical resection is possible.

PET

This is especially useful for detecting metastatic deposits. If curative surgical resection is to be considered, a PET scan can help to confirm that there is no distal metastatic spread prior to surgery.

CEA

Tumour markers can be used to determine the effectiveness of treatment and to assess for disease recurrence. CEA also has a prognostic role, with higher levels corresponding to a poorer prognosis. Tumour markers have no role in the diagnosis of a malignancy.

Staging of colorectal cancer is based on the TNM classification (*see* Table 12.1), which has largely superseded the Dukes staging system.

TABLE 12.1 TNM staging system for colorectal cancer

STAGE	PRIMARY TUMOUR (T)	REGIONAL LYMPH NODE (N)	REMOTE METASTASIS (M)
Stage 0	Carcinoma *in situ* (Tis)	N0	M0
Stage I	Tumour may invade sub-mucosa (T1) or muscularis propria (T2)	N0	M0
Stage II	Tumour invades muscularis (T3) or adjacent organs or structures (T4)	N0	M0
Stage IIA	T3	N0	M0
Stage IIB	T4a	N0	M0
Stage IIC	T4b	N0	M0
Stage IIIA	T1–4	N1–2	M0
Stage IIIB	T1–4	N1–2	M0
Stage IIIC	T3–4	N1–2	M0
Stage IVA	T1–4	N1–3	M1a
Stage IVB	T1–4	N1–3	M1b

Management
Medical management
Radiotherapy is useful for patients with stage II and stage III disease.

Chemotherapy
Chemotherapy in the form of fluorouracil has been demonstrated to be beneficial in patients with stage III disease. Palliative chemotherapy is used for patients with metastatic disease. Agents such as irinotecan or oxaliplatin have shown worthwhile survival response rates.

Radiotherapy
Radiotherapy is commonly used in patients with rectal disease. However, this may result in radiation proctitis, causing PR bleeding which can be difficult to control. The main role of radiotherapy in colorectal cancer is in palliative treatment of metastatic disease (usually in brain and bone).

Nutrition
The combination of the catabolic state of malignancy and poor appetite results in malnutrition. Assessment of the patient by a dietician can help to stabilise their weight, and is important in pre-operative optimisation.

Novel therapies
Trials that are currently in progress have demonstrated promising results with the use of antibodies directed against vascular endothelial growth factor and epidermal growth factor receptor (e.g. bevacizumab and cetuximab, respectively).

Surgical management
Surgery is the mainstay of therapy for localised stage I, II and III colorectal cancer. Total mesorectal excision is now being employed for rectal cancer, as it has been shown to reduce recurrence and peri-operative morbidity. Fast-track surgery, whereby urinary catheters, drains and nasogastric tubes are avoided, enables a reduction in hospital stay and peri-operative morbidity.

Laparoscopic surgery is often utilised in the treatment of colorectal cancer. Sentinel lymph node mapping is useful for patients with stage II disease, and allows clinicians to determine which lymph nodes have the highest risk of harbouring metastatic disease.

Daily monitoring/investigations
1 Close observation of vital signs.

2   Daily examination, looking specifically for signs of abdominal tenderness which raise the possibility of perforation or obstruction.
3   FBC, U&Es, CRP, LFTs and clotting twice per week.

Important tips

Multidisciplinary team
Colorectal cancer requires management by a multidisciplinary team, which will consist of gastroenterologists, colorectal surgeons, oncologists, specialist nurses and dieticians.

Post-operative screening
Patients must undergo screening colonoscopy for disease recurrence 1 year post surgery. Colonoscopy must then be repeated every 3 years thereafter, unless recurrence is suspected before this.

Screening
Patients with a family history of high-risk conditions, especially HNPCC and FAP, must be enrolled in a screening programme.

Palliative care
Confirmed cases of colorectal cancer should be discussed with a palliative care team. The prognosis for colorectal cancer is extremely poor, and good-quality management of symptoms is essential for the patient and their family. In cases where curative resection is to be undertaken, the palliative care team may also have a useful role in the control of pain and nausea/vomiting.

Information to have to hand for ward rounds
1   Up-to-date bloods, including FBC, U&Es, LFTs and CEA.
2   The results of the most recent colonoscopy, or the date when it is booked.
3   Knowledge of comorbidities, family history and the patient's functional status, as this will affect possible management options.
4   Staging CT report, or the date when it is booked.
5   Observation chart for temperature and haemodynamic status.

Further reading
- Steward BW and Kleihues P, eds. Colorectal cancer. In: *World Cancer Report*. Lyon: IARC Press; 2003. pp. 198–202.

- Sobin LH and Wittekind C, eds. *TNM Classification of Malignant Tumours*, 6th edn. New York: Wiley-Liss; 2002.
- Andre T, Boni C, Mounedji-Boudiaf L *et al.* Oxaliplatin, fluorouracil, and leucovorin as adjuvant treatment for colon cancer. *New England Journal of Medicine* 2004; **350**: 2343–51.
- Hurwitz H, Fehrenbacher L, Novotny W *et al.* Bevacizumab plus irinotecan, fluorouracil, and leucovorin for metastatic colorectal cancer. *New England Journal of Medicine* 2004; **350**: 2335–42.
- Cunningham D, Humblet Y, Siena S *et al.* Cetuximab monotherapy and cetuximab plus irinotecan in irinotecan-refractory metastatic colorectal cancer. *New England Journal of Medicine* 2004; **351**: 337–45.
- Cecil TD, Sexton R, Moran BJ *et al.* Total mesorectal excision results in low local recurrence rates in lymph node-positive rectal cancer. *Diseases of the Colon and Rectum* 2004; **47**: 1145–50.
- Kehlet H and Dahl JB. Anaesthesia, surgery, and challenges in postoperative recovery. *Lancet* 2003; **362**: 1921–8.
- Clinical Outcomes of Surgical Therapy Study Group. A comparison of laparoscopically assisted and open colectomy for colon cancer. *New England Journal of Medicine* 2004; **350**: 2050–59.
- Saha S, Dan AG, Beutler T *et al.* Sentinel lymph node mapping technique in colon cancer. *Seminars in Oncology* 2004; **31**: 374–81.

13

Jaundice

Jaundice is usually detectable when the serum bilirubin concentration is
> 35 mmol/l.

Jaundice can be classified in many different ways. It is commonly divided
into three categories on the basis of bilirubin metabolism, namely pre-
hepatic jaundice, hepatocellular jaundice and cholestatic jaundice. However,
in clinical practice patients may have a combination of all three types.

Bilirubin metabolism

Bilirubin is formed by the breakdown of haemoglobin in the spleen. It
is then conjugated with glucoronic acid in hepatocytes to become water
soluble. This water-soluble conjugated bilirubin is secreted into the bile and
enters the small intestine. Approximately 80% of it enters the enterohepatic
circulation (i.e. is taken up again by the liver), and the rest is converted to
urobilinogen by intestinal bacteria. Urobilinogen that remains in the gut is
either reabsorbed through the gut wall or converted to stercobilin, which is
responsible for the brown colour of faeces.

Aetiology

Pre-hepatic jaundice

Disorders that lead to pre-hepatic jaundice are caused by excessive production of bilirubin in the spleen. Unconjugated bilirubin enters the blood
bound to albumin, which is insoluble in water, so it is not excreted in the
urine. Pre-hepatic jaundice is detected by the finding of raised unconjugated (indirect) bilirubin levels in the blood. Common causes include the
following:

- neonatal jaundice
- haemolysis

- Gilbert's syndrome (glucuronyl transferase deficiency)
- dyserythropoiesis.

Hepatocellular jaundice

This type of jaundice develops when hepatocytes are damaged, usually by diffuse injury or inflammation. This is detected by the finding of raised conjugated (direct) bilirubin levels in the blood. Causes include the following:
- viruses (e.g. CMV, EBV, hepatitis A, B, C, D and E)
- cirrhosis (scarring of the hepatocytes, which is the end result of chronic inflammation of any aetiology)
- alcoholic hepatitis
- autoimmune hepatitis (AIH)
- drug induced (e.g. paracetamol, isoniazid, rifampicin, statins)
- blockage of the portal vein (Budd–Chiari syndrome)
- failure to excrete conjugated bilirubin (Dubin–Johnson syndrome)
- right heart failure.

Cholestatic jaundice (obstructive jaundice)

Cholestatic jaundice occurs when the common bile duct (CBD) becomes blocked. Conjugated bilirubin is therefore reabsorbed into the blood, and less of it enters the gut, leading to reduced stercobilin levels in the stools, which are therefore lighter in colour. The water-soluble conjugated bilirubin is excreted in the urine, causing it to darken. Causes of cholestatic jaundice include the following:
- gallstones in the CBD
- pancreatic cancer (compressing the CBD)
- primary biliary cirrhosis (damage to interlobar bile ducts by chronic granulomatous inflammation)
- lymph nodes at the porta hepatis
- cholangiocarcinoma (cancer of the bile ducts)
- sclerosing cholangitis (scarring of the bile ducts)
- drugs (e.g. co-amoxiclav).

Levels of both the conjugated and unconjugated fractions of bilirubin in the blood may be raised in any cause of chronic liver disease.

Clinical presentation

History

A full medical history is required in all patients who present with jaundice. It is important to enquire about the following in particular:
- **occupation:** industrial exposure to hepatoxic agents or use of alcohol

- **travel abroad:** visit to an area where viral hepatitis is endemic, or contact with malaria
- **contact with jaundiced patients:** hepatitis A is spread by the faeco-oral route, whereas hepatitis B and C are bloodborne viruses (BBV)
- **presence of tattoos and body piercing:** BBV risk
- **previous blood transfusions:** BBV risk
- **alcohol consumption:** alcoholic hepatitis and cirrhosis
- **medication use:** ask about over-the-counter medication, herbal supplements and recreational drugs (including anabolic steroids)
- **sexual history:** BBV risk
- **family history:** vertical and childhood transmission of hepatitis B and C; autoimmune conditions may be inherited
- **pregnancy**
- **other medical problems.**

Examination
A full system examination should be performed. Signs that may be elicited include the following:
- **tremulousness and sweating:** alcohol withdrawal
- **fevers and rigors:** infection (e.g. hepatic abscess, cholangitis)
- **weight loss:** malignancy, chronic liver disease
- **lethargy, irritability, confusion or reduced GCS score:** these signs may suggest hepatic encephalopathy, or alcohol intoxication or withdrawal
- **lymphadenopathy:** malignancy or infection
- **tender hepatomegaly:** this may be found in acute causes of jaundice
- **palpable gallbladder:** Courvoisier's law states that in the presence of a palpable gallbladder, painless jaundice is unlikely to be caused by gallstones. Gallstones usually develop slowly over time and therefore result in a shrunken, fibrotic, poorly distensible gallbladder. The gallbladder tends to be enlarged in pathologies that cause obstruction of the biliary tree over a shorter period of time (e.g. pancreatic cancer)
- **examination of the urine and stools:** pale stools and dark urine are a sign of obstructive jaundice.
  In particular, note any evidence of chronic liver disease:
- **palmar erythema:** signs of a hyperdynamic circulation
- **caput medusa:** portal hypertension leads to the development of porto-systemic collateral channels. Abdominal wall collateral veins may appear as vessels that radiate out from the umbilicus
- **ascites:** the impaired hepatic metabolism of endogenous vasodilators leads to peripheral vasodilatation. This causes decreased renal blood flow and the stimulation of the renin–angiotensin–aldosterone axis

with salt and water retention. At least 1500 ml of ascitic fluid must be present for detection by clinical examination, whereas ultrasound can detect much smaller volumes (≤ 500 ml). Ascites may be categorised as follows:

— **Grade 1 – mild ascites:** this is only detectable by ultrasound examination.
— **Grade 2 – moderate ascites:** this causes moderate symmetrical distension of the abdomen.
— **Grade 3 – large ascites:** this causes marked abdominal distension

- **splenomegaly:** secondary to portal hypertension
- **spider naevi:** a central arteriole from which numerous small branches radiate; they blanch when the lesions are compressed. They most often occur in the upper trunk. The pathogenesis is unclear, but is thought to be related to raised oestradiol levels which are a result of reduced breakdown of androstenedione by the liver
- **purpura:** coagulopathy may develop in the presence of severe liver damage, due to clotting factor deficiency
- **gynaecomastia:** this is caused by reduced liver catabolism of androstenedione, which increases oestrogen precursors and plasma levels of oestradiol. The resulting increase in the ratio of free oestradiol to free testosterone causes feminisation. The use of spironolactone as a treatment for ascites may also contribute to gynaecomastia, as it is an inhibitor of testosterone synthesis
- **altered pattern of body hair:** as above
- **pruritus:** this is a common complaint in chronic liver disease. The pathogenesis is unclear, but it may be related to bile acid accumulation. Bile acid binding agents are traditionally used as treatment, with varying degrees of success
- **asterixis:** this is related to raised ammonia levels. Ammonia is a degradation product of the intestinal flora that has neurotoxic effects. It is cleared by the liver, and may accumulate in liver failure
- **encephalopathy:** this is a neuropsychiatric complication of liver failure. It is defined as a disturbance in central nervous function due to hepatic insufficiency, and is related to raised ammonia levels. It is characterised by a change in personality and intellect, and a depressed level of consciousness. The grading of encephalopathy is summarised in Table 13.1.

TABLE 13.1 Grading of encephalopathy

GRADE	SYMPTOMS	SIGNS	GCS SCORE
1	Short attention span	Tremor Ataxia Incoordination	15
2	Lethargy Disorientation Personality change	Asterixis Ataxia Dysarthria	11–15
3	Confusion Somnolence	Asterixis Ataxia	8–11
4	Coma	Decerebration	< 8

Initial investigations

- **FBC.** Neutrophilia may suggest infection. Thrombocytopaenia may occur in chronic liver disease as a result of functional hyposplenism.
- **Blood film and reticulocyte count.** Films may show polychromasia, spherocytes, macrocytosis and fragmented cells in jaundice secondary to haemolysis. The percentage of reticulocytes present will also be increased. Serum LDH levels may also be raised, and serum haptoglobin levels are low in haemolysis.
- **Coombs' test (direct antihuman globulin).** This is positive in immune-mediated haemolytic anaemia.
- **U&Es.** Hyponatraemia may occur in secondary aldosteronism secondary to cirrhosis. A disproportionately low creatinine concentration may reflect low body mass in a patient with a history of chronic alcohol use. Urea levels are frequently low due to poor nutritional status.
- **LFTs.** ALT, AST, ALP, GGT, albumin, total protein and bilirubin (direct and indirect) should be checked. A disproportionate rise in transaminase activity occurs in hepatitis, whereas ALP activity is disproportionately high in cholestatic liver disease.
- **Clotting factors.** INR is the best marker of liver synthetic function, and you must pay particular attention to this. The INR provides a marker of the severity of impairment of synthetic liver function and can also be used as a guide to deterioration or improvement of a patient's condition.
- **Viral serologies.** IgM anti-HAV, HBsAg, IgM anti-HBc, anti-HCV and anti-HEV should be checked.
- **Autoantibodies.** Anti-nuclear antibodies (ANA) and anti-smooth muscle antibodies (ASMA) may be positive in chronic active hepatitis,

and AMA (anti-mitochondrial antibodies) may be positive in primary biliary cirrhosis.

- **Blood cultures.** These are required to exclude infection.
- **Paracetamol level and toxicology screen.** These are needed to test for drug-induced hepatitis.
- **ABGs and lactic acid.** These may indicate and establish the severity of shock associated with liver failure.
- **Ammonia.** Levels may be raised in hepatic encephalopathy. Contact the biochemistry lab before this sample is taken, as it requires advance preparation.
- **CXR.** This is required to rule out infection. Depending on the level of hypoalbuminaemia, the patient may have pleural effusions.
- **Abdominal US with Dopplers of the portal vein and hepatic vessels.** Bile duct dilation may occur in extrahepatic jaundice, a small shrunken liver suggests cirrhosis, and the presence of masses may suggest primary or metastatic cancer, hepatomas or abscesses. It is important to check that the blood supply to the liver is intact by imaging the portal and hepatic veins.
- **Pregnancy test.** This should be performed in all women of childbearing age.

Further investigations

Copper profile

This is useful if it is suspected that the patient may have Wilson's disease, which is an autosomal recessive genetic disorder that results in the accumulation of copper in the liver and brain. It can be manifested by a variety of neuropsychiatric symptoms, or by signs and symptoms of liver disease. It is detected by demonstrating reduced blood copper and caeruloplasmin levels and elevated 24-hour urinary copper excretion. Liver biopsy and molecular genetic testing are used to confirm the diagnosis.

Iron profile

This is useful if haemochromatosis is suspected. This is an autosomal recessive disorder of iron metabolism whereby increased amounts of iron absorbed from the intestine are deposited in the liver, heart and endocrine glands. It may be detected by abnormal LFTs, raised serum ferritin levels, raised serum iron levels, reduced total iron-binding capacity (TIBC) and a transferrin saturation of > 80%. A liver biopsy and HFE gene mutation testing are diagnostic.

Alphafetoprotein

This may be raised in the presence of primary or secondary malignancy in the liver.

Diagnostic paracentesis

Urgent microscopy and culture is needed to exclude spontaneous bacterial peritonitis (SBP). This occurs in 10–30% of patients with ascites, and has a mortality rate of 20%. The patient may be asymptomatic, and a diagnostic paracentesis is mandatory in all patients with cirrhosis who require hospitalisation. The usual organisms cultured in the case of SBP are *E. coli*, streptococci and enterococci. Antibiotics should be started if the ascitic fluid has a white cell count of >250 cells/mm^3.

Interpretation of liver function tests

ALT and AST are two sensitive markers of hepatocellular injury or necrosis. ALT is the more specific of the two enzymes for liver damage, as it is chiefly present in the cytosol of the liver cell, whereas AST has both cytosolic and mitochondrial forms, and may be found in liver, heart, skeletal muscle, kidneys, brain, pancreas, lungs and blood cells. However, both ALT and AST may be normal even in the presence of severe liver damage, as necrosed hepatocytes do not release further enzymes. The ALT/AST ratio may sometimes be useful for differentiating between causes of liver damage.

- A ratio of > 2 is associated with alcoholic hepatitis.
- A ratio of < 1 is associated with viral hepatitis.
- A ratio ≤ 1 is associated with acute and chronic liver injury or steatosis (fatty infiltration of the liver).

Raised serum ALP and GGT activity may be found in any hepatobiliary pancreatic disease. GGT is more specific for liver disease than ALP, as the latter may also be raised in bone disorders. Isolated elevation or disproportionate elevation of GGT activity compared with the other liver enzymes may indicate alcohol abuse or alcoholic liver disease.

High activity of GGT and ALP may suggest bile duct damage or blockage (cholestasis). Intrahepatic cholestasis refers to bile duct blockage or injury within the liver (e.g. primary biliary cirrhosis). Extrahepatic cholestasis refers to bile duct blockage or injury that occurs outside the liver (e.g. gallstones).

TABLE 13.2 Interpretation of liver function tests

TEST	NORMAL	PREHEPATIC	HEPATOCELLULAR	EXTRAHEPATIC
Bilirubin (μmol/l)	< 17	50–150	50–400	100–900
AST (IU/l)	< 35	< 35	300–10 000	35–400
ALP (IU/l)	< 120	< 120	120–300	> 300
GGT (IU/l)	15–40	15–40	15–200	80–1000
Albumin (g/dl)	4–5	4–5	2–5	3–5
Hb (g/dl)	12–16	< 10	12–16	10–16
Reticulocytes (%)	< 1	10–30	< 1	< 1
INR	1.1–1.2	1.0–1.2	1.0–30 +	1.0–3.0 (falls in response to IV vitamin K)

Management

The management of jaundice depends on its cause. The most common presentations to hospital in the UK are the result of alcoholic hepatitis, decompensated cirrhosis of all aetiologies, and common bile duct stones.

Alcoholic hepatitis

This may present with jaundice, fever, tender hepatomegaly and signs of alcohol withdrawal.

1 Obtain senior help early on, as the mortality rate is up to 30%.
2 Many patients will require chlordiazepoxide or benzodiazepines to prevent the symptoms of withdrawal and reduce the risk of delirium tremens.
3 Calculate the severity of presentation by using Maddrey's discriminate function for alcoholic hepatitis. An index of > 32 indicates a severe attack with a 30-day mortality rate of 35–45%. These patients may benefit from steroids *after* infection has been excluded. The discriminant function is calculated using the following formula:

$$\text{patient's PT (seconds)} - \text{control PT} + \text{bilirubin} /17.1.$$

4 Dietary supplements – these patients are often malnourished and benefit from oral supplements or NG feeding. Ask for an urgent dietetic assessment. Dietary supplementation is the only measure that has been demonstrated to reduce mortality in acute alcoholic hepatitis.
5 The chronic drinker is likely to be deficient in vitamins A, B and C and folate. Give IV replacement for 3 days to replace these before switching to oral vitamins. Administration of Pabrinex 1 and 2 twice daily IV combined with thiamine 200 mg twice daily is advisable initially.

6 Strict fluid balance, stool and food charts should be maintained.

Decompensated cirrhosis (any aetiology)

Cirrhosis is the end stage of chronic inflammation and scarring of the liver, and is irreversible. Liver transplantation is the only cure. Patients with cirrhosis may deteriorate (decompensate) for a number of reasons (see below). Decompensation refers to the onset of one or more of jaundice, ascites, encephalopathy or coagulopathy in a patient with chronic liver disease.

1 Obtain senior help early on.
2 Assess the prognosis of the disease. A number of different scoring systems are available, including the Child–Pugh score and the MELD score (*see* Chapter 15).
3 Exclude precipitants, including GI bleeds, constipation, sedatives, infections (particularly spontaneous bacterial peritonitis if ascites is present) and alcohol use.
4 Monitor the patient daily for evidence of encephalopathy.
5 Patients with ascites may require a diagnostic or therapeutic drain.
6 Patients with liver disease appear to be particularly sensitive to sedatives, so always take senior advice if you feel that these may be required.
7 Give a proton pump inhibitor (PPI) for GI bleed prophylaxis.
8 In a patient with known portal hypertension and established varices secondary to cirrhosis, consider using a beta-blocker (e.g. propranolol 40 mg twice a day), as this will reduce the risk of variceal bleeding.
9 Ensure optimisation of nutrition with supplements and NG feeding if required.
10 A low-salt diet may help to prevent the accumulation of ascites.
11 Strict fluid balance – replacement fluid in established cirrhosis is contentious. Many specialised liver units recommend the use of colloids such as Gelofusine or human albumin solution (HAS). Normal saline was traditionally avoided, as it was thought to worsen the secondary hyperaldosteronism that develops in many patients with cirrhosis. However, this view is now largely obsolete. Dextrose 5% is not recommended, as it accumulates rapidly in the patient's third space and leaves them intravascularly depleted.
12 Consider the use of prophylactic antibiotics.
13 Laxatives – ensure that there are at least two daily bowel movements as monitored by a stool chart.

Common bile duct stones

Most gallstones are asymptomatic within the gallbladder, but cause symptoms if they become lodged in the gallbladder neck, the cystic duct or the common bile duct. This may lead to acute or chronic cholecystitis, which presents with right upper quadrant pain, fever, rigors and raised inflammatory markers.

1　Perform a USS to identify the presence of gallstones and assess for common bile duct (CBD) and intrahepatic bile duct dilatation.
2　Perform an AXR and look for visible stones. An erect CXR will help to exclude free air indicating perforation.
3　Prescribe intravenous antibiotics according to your local trust guidelines.
4　Endoscopic retrograde cholangiopancreatography (ERCP) is used to both diagnose and treat biliary obstruction. Magnetic resonance cholangiopancreatography (MRCP) is a non-invasive method of imaging the bile ducts, and may be used as the first-line investigation in some patients.
5　Surgery – consult the surgeons as soon as the diagnosis is suspected. Different surgeons will operate at different times in the course of acute cholecystitis.

Daily monitoring/investigations

1　Close observation of vital signs.
2　Daily review of the patient's clinical condition, and stool and fluid balance charts.
3　Daily examination, looking specifically for evidence of infection and decompensated liver disease. Score the patient's encephalopathy grade.
4　Daily bloods, including FBC, U&Es, LFTs and clotting if deranged initially.

Important tips

Diagnostic ascitic aspirate

Send the ascitic fluid samples marked as urgent. It is particularly important to phone the laboratory and warn them to expect a sample, and ask them to process the cell count and Gram stain as urgent. The results should be available within a couple of hours, and may guide your management in the case of SBP.

Radiology

Always perform an abdominal USS urgently in patients who present with jaundice. If there is biliary dilatation you must provide the patient with antibiotic cover according to your local trust guidelines, and contact the surgeons. Liver Doppler studies will also be beneficial in patients with suspected cirrhosis and acute portal vein thrombosis.

History

Documentation of a full medical, alcohol, sexual and drug history is extremely important in the context of a jaundiced patient. Specifically ask the patient whether they have:

- injected drugs or shared needles
- had casual sexual partners without using protection against sexually transmitted diseases
- had a blood transfusion, or any tattoos or piercings
- used herbal medications
- been in contact with a jaundiced individual.

In addition, take a comprehensive travel history. This must include location, stopovers en route, and use of malarial prophylaxis (if appropriate) and appropriate vaccinations for travel.

Microbiology

Patients with a source of infection, or a suspected source, should undergo a full septic screen. Any results should be closely followed up and treated appropriately in accordance with local antibiotic/antiviral guidelines. Discussion with a microbiologist may be advisable in complicated cases or those that are not responding appropriately to current treatments.

Cannulas

Intravenous cannulas are a common source of infection in hospitals. Ensure that you change the cannula every 3 days, and inspect cannula sites daily for early signs of local infection. Write the date of insertion on the cannula dressing, and record this in the notes to avoid confusion. If your patient is likely to require a prolonged course of antibiotics, you may wish to consider using a peripherally inserted central catheter (PICC) line.

Previous records

Review the patient's case notes, particularly for details of previous liver USS, OGD (especially in the context of patients with cirrhosis and known varices), and any previous episodes of jaundice or SBP.

Further advice

The family contacts of patients with viral hepatitis may need to be screened by their general practitioner.

Information to have to hand for ward rounds

1   Up-to-date blood results, including FBC, U&Es, LFTs, albumin and INR.

2 A copy of the US abdomen report.
3 The results of the liver database, including viral and autoimmune screens.
4 Up-to-date microbiology results.
5 The dates or results of further investigations, in particular the CT abdomen, ERCP and ascitic tap results.

14

Acute liver failure

Liver failure may occur suddenly in a previously healthy liver (acute), or as a consequence of chronic liver disease (acute on chronic liver failure).

The term *acute liver failure* (*ALF*) is used to describe the development of coagulopathy (INR > 1.5) and any degree of mental alteration (encephalopathy) in a patient without pre-existing cirrhosis and with an illness of less than 26 weeks' duration. Liver failure in the acute setting has a worse prognosis.

TABLE 14.1 Categories of acute liver failure

ACUTE LIVER FAILURE	JAUNDICE TO ENCEPHALOPATHY INTERVAL
Hyperacute hepatic failure	7 days
Fulminant hepatic failure	8 weeks
Sub-fulminant hepatic failure	26 weeks

Aetiology

- Infections (e.g. viral hepatitis A, B, C, D and E).
- Drugs (e.g. paracetamol). This is the commonest cause of liver failure in the UK. Ingestion of > 10 g paracetamol/24 hours, and of smaller doses in patients with alcoholic liver disease, may be hepatotoxic. Hepatotoxic drug effects may be dose related (those that will occur in most patients given a sufficiently high dose) or idiosyncratic drug reactions (unusual or unpredictable reactions), which usually occur within 6 months of starting the medication. As paracetamol is such a common aetiological factor, you should be familiar with the features of severe paracetamol toxicity, which are as follows:
  — rapid development of grade 2 encephalopathy
  — PT > 20 seconds at 24 hours, > 45 seconds at 48 hours, or > 50 seconds at 72 hours

- bilirubin concentration > 300 μmol/l
- falling plasma phosphate levels
- arterial pH < 7.3 more than 24 hours after ingestion
- creatinine concentration > 300 μmol/l
- age < 10 years or > 40 years.

- Ischaemic hepatitis may occur after prolonged hypotension (e.g. septic shock, cardiac arrest).
- Budd–Chiari syndrome is due to acute hepatic vein thrombosis, and typically occurs in women aged 20–40 years. Patients present with RUQ pain, hepatomegaly and ascites. Suspect an underlying haematological disorder (e.g. polycythaemia rubra vera) or other cause of thrombophilia. Diagnosis is by duplex ultrasound of the hepatic veins and inferior vena cava (IVC).

Clinical presentation

The wide variation in clinical presentation of liver failure of different aetiologies is beyond the scope of this book. Some general features can be applied when dividing patients into the crude categories of acute and chronic liver failure. These are summarised below.

Acute liver failure

There may be a 'flu-like' prodrome, especially in the case of acute viral infection. Patients will not have manifestations of chronic liver disease such as spider naevi, palmar erythema, caput medusa, etc., but are more likely to be encephalopathic, jaundiced, and have tender hepatomegaly with or without ascites. Complications of ALF can include the following:

- bleeding
- infection
- ascites
- hypoglycaemia
- cerebral oedema
- hepatorenal syndrome.

Chronic liver failure

These patients will often have a shrunken, cirrhotic liver that is not palpable. Ascites may or may not be present. There may be evidence of chronic liver failure (e.g. spider naevi, hair loss and gynaecomastia).

Initial investigations

- **FBC.** There may not be changes to the FBC in the acute setting. There may be a lymphocytosis in the context of viral infection. Normocytic anaemia may represent haemolysis.

- **Blood film and reticulocyte count, serum LDH and serum haptoglobin levels.** These may be useful if coexisting haemolysis is suspected.
- **U&Es.** Renal function may be impaired in some causes of ALF, and is particularly important in paracetamol overdose.
- **Serum glucose level.** Hypoglycaemia in the context of paracetamol overdose is a marker of severe liver impairment.
- **LFTs.** Either a cholestatic or hepatitic picture may be observed. Hypoalbuminaemia may represent poor synthetic function.
- **Coagulation factors.** PT and INR are markers of synthetic liver function.
- **Group and save.**
- **ABG.** pH is an important marker of severity in acute liver failure, and makes up part of the King's College Hospital Criteria for liver transplantation. A pH of < 7.3 in a patient with paracetamol overdose is by itself an indication for referral for liver transplant.
- **Viral serology.** This should include IgM anti-HAV, HBsAg, IgM anti-HBc, anti-HCV, anti-HEV and HIV (the patient's consent is required for the latter).
- **Autoantibodies.** These should include ANA, AMA, ASMA and immunoglobulins.
- **Cultures.** These should include blood, urine, stool and sputum.
- **Paracetamol level and toxicology screen.**
- **Plasma caeruloplasmin.**
- **CXR.** This is needed as part of the septic screen, and may reveal pleural effusions in the context of hypoalbuminaemia.

Further investigations
USS
Imaging of the liver architecture and for focal liver lesions can be undertaken with ultrasound. Doppler studies of the portal vein and hepatic vessels should also be performed in order to exclude thrombus.

Diagnostic paracentesis
A sample of ascitic fluid should be obtained. Draw off approximately 20–50 ml of ascitic fluid and send it urgently for an MC&S. The sample should also be sent for cytology and biochemical analysis. Spontaneous bacterial peritonitis should be empirically treated if the ascitic WCC is > 250 cells/mm^3.

Management
General management

- Obtain senior help early on. These patients can be extremely unwell, and may require advanced management by a specialist in a specialist centre.
- Intensive care or high dependency unit nursing will be required.
- Ensure that the patient's airway is protected (go through the usual ABCDE method of assessment, as with any sick patient).
- Insert a central line early on to ensure that an accurate assessment of fluid balance can be made. Two large-bore peripheral venous access sites should also be sought.
- Monitor temperature, pulse, blood pressure, urine output, blood glucose and sedation score on an hourly basis.
- Maintain fluid and electrolyte balance. Keep the potassium concentration > 3.5 mmol/l. Consider the use of human albumin solution after discussion with a gastroenterology registrar or consultant.
- Give a proton pump inhibitor (PPI) for GI bleed prophylaxis.
- Reassess the patient daily for evidence of encephalopathy and ascites, and to monitor fluid balance.
- Avoid using sedatives if possible.
- Ensure optimisation of nutrition with supplements and NG feeding if required. Aim for a protein intake of 60 g/day.
- Vitamin supplementation – it is especially important to administer thiamine and Pabrinex early in the course of the patient's presentation.
- Laxatives – ensure that there are at least two daily bowel movements. Often lactulose 30 ml is given 4-hourly.
- Consider liver transplantation, and discuss this with a transplant centre.
- If encephalopathy is grade 2 or higher, or if the systolic blood pressure is < 90 mmHg, site central venous and radial arterial lines. Check the platelet count and clotting screen before performing any invasive procedure.
- If encephalopathy is grade 3 or higher, arrange elective intubation and ventilation.

Prescribing N-acetyl cysteine (NAC) in paracetamol overdose

1 Take a full history in any case of suspected overdose, including the time of ingestion, whether the overdose was staggered (i.e. whether it took place over several hours or days), the quantity of any medication taken, use of recreational drugs or over-the-counter medications, and alcohol ingestion (both chronically and acutely).

2 The *British National Formulary* (*BNF*) and most Accident and Emergency departments will have a treatment threshold in the paracetamol

poisoning monograph. This triages patients into high and normal risk. Treat patients with chronic alcohol abuse, chronic malnutrition or recent starvation, HIV/AIDS or patients on hepatic enzyme inducers (phenytoin, carbamazepine, barbituates, rifampicin, alcohol, sulphonylureas) as high risk.

3 Start NAC immediately if the patient has ingested > 150 mg/kg or > 12 g of paracetamol.
4 Check the plasma paracetamol level at 4 hours post-ingestion.
5 Start NAC infusion at this stage if the patient meets the treatment criteria.
6 Stop NAC if the plasma paracetamol level at > 4 hours post-ingestion is below the treatment line, unless there is a risk of staggered poisoning.
7 Prescribe NAC on the fluid chart, and inform the nursing staff.
8 Consider checking the salicylate level.

Acetyl cysteine replenishes mitochondrial and cytosolic glutathione. Oral methionine can be used for patients who are allergic to NAC. Minor reactions to NAC can occur (e.g. flushing, pruritus, urticaria). If there is a severe reaction, stop the infusion and give an antihistamine (e.g. chlorphenamine 10 mg IV over 10 minutes).

Management of specific complications in acute liver failure
Bleeding
- Vitamin K 10 mg IV once a day for 2–3 days.
- Platelet transfusion if platelet count is $< 50 \times 10^9/l$.
- Fresh frozen plasma (FFP) if the prothrombin time (PT) is > 20 seconds and/or APTT is > 48 seconds (e.g. 10–15 ml/kg, or 4 units).
- Blood transfusion if haemoglobin concentration is < 10 g/dl. Caution is needed in patients with variceal bleeding, as over-transfusion might precipitate further bleeding.

Ascites
- Diagnostic ascitic fluid aspiration to exclude SBP (send for an urgent cell count and Gram staining).
- Fluid restriction.
- Low-salt diet.
- Diuretics (e.g. furosemide 40 mg once a day with spironolactone 100 mg once a day).
- Daily weights (aim for a weight loss of 0.5 kg/day).
- Therapeutic paracentesis if there is tense ascites (see Chapter 3).

Infection
- Culture urine, stool, ascites, blood, stool and sputum.

- Liaise with a microbiologist. You may need empirical antibiotics in accordance with local trust guidelines.
- Avoid using nephrotoxic antimicrobial agents (e.g. gentamicin).

Hypoglycaemia
- Monitor blood sugar levels frequently (e.g. 2-hourly).
- Maintain Boehringer Mannheim (BM) > 3.5 mmol/l.
- Treat with 50 ml of 50% dextrose if BM is < 2 mmol/l.

Cerebral oedema
- Do not manage this alone. These patients must be urgently discussed with your seniors and managed in an intensive care setting.
- 20% mannitol IV should be administered under specialist supervision only.
- Patients are likely to require intubation and hyperventilation to induce a respiratory alkalosis in an attempt to reduce intracranial pressure.
- An intercranial pressure (ICP) bolt may be required. This device should only be inserted by a neurosurgeon.

Hepatorenal syndrome (HRS)
HRS occurs in approximately 10% of patients with cirrhosis and ascites, and has a high mortality. Deteriorating liver function leads to renal vasoconstriction and renal impairment.

All patients who develop HRS and who are transplant candidates should be considered for transplantation at this stage. Two forms of hepatorenal syndrome have been identified (*see* Table 14.2).
- Type 1 HRS is characterised by rapidly progressive renal failure, with a doubling of serum creatinine concentration to > 221 μmol/l (2.5 mg/dl), or a halving of the creatinine clearance to < 20 ml/minute over a period of less than 2 weeks. The mortality rate for type 1 HRS is over 50% at 1 month.
- Type 2 HRS is slower in onset and progression. It is defined by an increase in serum creatinine concentration to > 133 μmol/l (1.5 mg/dl), or a creatinine clearance of < 40 ml/minute, and a urine sodium concentration of < 10 μmol/l. It has a median survival time of 6 months without liver transplantation.

It is vital to ensure that the patient is adequately hydrated in order to prevent renal failure. Human albumin solution (HAS) is often used as volume replacement in HRS alongside terlipressin (a vasopressin analogue), and may reduce mortality and improve renal function (e.g. HAS 20% 1 g/kg daily plus terlipressin 0.5 mg IV twice a day). Haemofiltration or dialysis is rarely used because the prognosis of established liver and renal failure is so poor.

TABLE 14.2 Characteristics of the two forms of hepatorenal syndrome (HRS)

	HRS 1	HRS 2
Onset	Within 2 weeks	Gradual
Serum creatinine concentration	> 221 µmol/l	> 133 µmol/l
Creatinine clearance	< 20 ml/min	< 40 ml/min
Urine sodium concentration		< 10 µmol/l

Diagnosis of HRS: major and minor criteria
Major criteria
These are liver disease and renal failure, in the absence of:
- shock
- infection
- recent exposure to nephrotoxic drugs
- fluid losses
- proteinuria
- renal disease or outflow tract obstruction
- sustained improvement in renal function despite treatment with 1.5 litres of intravenous normal saline.

Minor criteria
These are as follows:
- urine volume < 500 ml/day
- low urinary sodium concentration
- urine osmolality greater than blood osmolality
- no haematuria
- serum sodium concentration < 130 mmol/l.

Indications for hepatic transplantation
Unwell patients with liver failure should be discussed with the local transplant centre early in their admission.

The transplant survival rate in patients with ALF is 65% at 1 year.

The King's College Hospital Criteria for hepatic transplantation are listed in Table 14.3.

TABLE 14.3 King's College Hospital Criteria for hepatic transplantation

Paracetamol-induced	Arterial pH < 7.3
	or all of the following:
	PT (prothrombin time) > 100 seconds
	Creatinine concentration > 300 μmol/l
Non-paracetamol-induced	PT > 100 seconds
	or three out of five of the following:
	Drug-induced liver failure
	Age < 11 years or > 40 years
	> 7 days between the onset of jaundice and encephalopathy
	PT > 50 seconds
	Bilirubin concentration > 300 μmol/l

Daily monitoring/investigations

1 Close observation of vital signs.
2 Daily review of the patient's clinical condition, and stool and fluid balance charts.
3 Daily examination, looking specifically for evidence of infection, decompensation and encephalopathy.
4 Daily bloods, including FBC, U&Es, LFTs and clotting.

Important tips

Specialist advice

Patients with acute liver failure are extremely ill and difficult to manage. All of these patients should be discussed with your local liver unit or the gastroenterologists at an early stage.

Cannulas

Intravenous cannulas are a common source of infection in hospitals. Ensure that you change the cannula every 3 days, and inspect cannula sites daily for early signs of local infection. Write the date of insertion on the cannula dressing, and record this in the notes to avoid confusion. If your patient is likely to require a prolonged course of antibiotics, you may wish to consider using a peripherally inserted central catheter (PICC) line.

Previous records

Review the patient's case notes, particularly for details of previous admissions with any hepatic-related problems. Previous USS liver, OGD or clinic letters may be of benefit.

Information to have to hand for ward rounds

1. Up-to-date bloods, including FBC, U&Es, LFTs and clotting.
2. The results of hepatitis serology and viral screening.
3. The results of the most recent liver USS and Doppler.
4. Up-to-date microbiology results.
5. Observation chart for temperature and haemodynamic status.

Further reading

- Travis S, Ahmad T, Collier J *et al. Pocket Consultant Gastroenterology*, 3rd edn. Oxford: Wiley-Blackwell; 2005.
- Moore KP and Aithal GP. Guidelines on the management of ascites in cirrhosis. *Gut* 2006; **55 (Suppl. 6):** vi1–12.
- Ferenci P, Lockwood A, Mullen K *et al.* Hepatic encephalopathy – definition, nomenclature, diagnosis, and quantification: final report of the working party at the 11th World Congresses of Gastroenterology, Vienna, 1998. *Hepatology* 2002; **35:** 716–21.
- Carraceni P and Van Thiel DH. Acute liver failure. *Lancet* 1995; **345:** 163–9.
- Kamath PS, Wiesner RH, Malinchoc M *et al.* A model to predict survival in patients with end-stage liver disease. *Hepatology* 2001; **33:** 464–70.
- Arroyo V, Ginès P, Gerbes AL *et al.* Definition and diagnostic criteria of refractory ascites and hepatorenal syndrome in cirrhosis. International Ascites Club. *Hepatology* 1996; **23:** 164–76.

15

Cirrhosis

Cirrhosis is irreversible liver damage with the formation of fibrosis and nodular regeneration secondary to the loss of normal hepatic architecture. It may be the final stage of chronic liver disease of many causes.

Aetiology
Common causes
- Alcohol.
- Chronic viral hepatitis (B and C).
- Non-alcoholic fatty liver disease (NAFLD).

Uncommon causes
- Autoimmune cirrhosis.
- Cryptogenic cirrhosis.
- Primary biliary cirrhosis.
- Primary sclerosing cholangitis.

Rare causes
- Wilson's disease.
- Haemochromatosis.
- Alpha-1-antitrypsin deficiency.
- Drugs (e.g. methotrexate).
- Budd–Chiari syndrome – occlusion of hepatic veins.
- Right heart failure.
- Secondary biliary cirrhosis (e.g. sclerosing cholangitis, cystic fibrosis).

Clinical presentation

The patient may be asymptomatic at presentation. It is important to examine them for evidence of chronic liver disease and decompensation.

Stigmata of chronic liver disease

- Leukonychia.
- Palmar erythema – this is a sign of a hyperdynamic circulation.
- Clubbing.
- Spider naevi.
- Telangiectasia.
- Gynaecomastia.
- Testicular atrophy.
- Enlarged liver or small shrunken liver (advanced cirrhosis).
- Jaundice.

Stigmata of decompensated liver disease

- Ascites.
- Variceal bleeding.
- Spontaneous bacterial peritonitis.
- Hepatic encephalopathy (confusion, reduced GCS score, liver flap).
- Hepatorenal syndrome (a rapid deterioration in kidney function).

History

- Alcohol use – amount, frequency, and type of alcohol ingested, as well as length of time for which the patient has been drinking to excess. Do not accept 'social' alcohol intake as an answer. You must be specific. If alcohol misuse is a concern, the CAGE questionnaire may be a useful screening tool, and has been validated to identify alcoholism. Two 'yes' responses indicate that the respondent should be investigated further:
  1 Have you ever felt that you needed to Cut down on your drinking?
  2 Have people ever Annoyed you by criticising your drinking?
  3 Have you ever felt Guilty about your drinking?
  4 Have you ever felt that you needed a drink first thing in the morning (an Eye-opener) to steady your nerves or to get rid of a hangover?
- Drugs, including paracetamol, over-the-counter medication, recreational drugs and herbal remedies.
- Occupation.
- Blood transfusions prior to 1991, when screening for hepatitis C began.
- Intravenous drug use and high-risk sexual activity (viral hepatitis risk).
- History of tattoos (viral hepatitis risk).
- Travel history (viral hepatitis risk).

- Family history – inherited defects (e.g. haemochromatosis, vertical transmission of viral hepatitis).
- Drug use (e.g. methotrexate- and methyldopa-associated cirrhosis).
- Past medical history (e.g. ulcerative colitis associated with sclerosing cholangitis, diabetes mellitus, obesity and hyperlipidaemia associated with fatty liver disease).
- Evidence of decompensation (e.g. ascites, variceal bleeding and encephalopathy).

Hepatic encephalopathy should be graded according to the West Haven classification criteria (*see* Box 15.1). It is important to exclude potentially treatable precipitants. A raised blood ammonia level may be detected in some cases of encephalopathy. This test requires close liaison with the laboratory, as there are special requirements for performing the test.

BOX 15.1 West Haven grading of encephalopathy

- **Grade 0:** Minimal hepatic encephalopathy. Lack of detectable changes in personality or behaviour. Small changes in cognitive function and coordination.
- **Grade 1:** Asterixis may be detected. Minimal impairment of cognitive function (ask the patient to add or subtract). Altered sleep patterns. Changes in mood.
- **Grade 2:** Asterixis. Disorientation. Drowsiness. Clear deficits in cognitive function and personality changes.
- **Grade 3:** Asterixis. Somnolent, but can be aroused. Unable to perform mental tasks, disorientation in time and place, and confusion.
- **Grade 4:** Coma with or without response to painful stimuli.

Common precipitants of encephalopathy

1 **Renal failure:** this leads to decreased clearance of urea, ammonia and other nitrogenous compounds.
2 **Gastrointestinal bleeding:** this causes an increase in ammonia levels secondary to the breakdown of blood in the gut.
3 **Infection:** this may predispose to impaired renal function and increased tissue catabolism, both of which increase blood ammonia levels.
4 **Constipation:** this increases intestinal production and absorption of ammonia.
5 **Medications:** drugs that act upon the central nervous system may worsen encephalopathy.

6 **Diuretic therapy:** decreased serum potassium levels and alkalosis may facilitate the conversion of ammonium (NH_4^+) ions to ammonia (NH_3).

Initial investigations

- **FBC.** Normocytic anaemia of chronic disease may occur. A low WCC may occur as a result of bone-marrow suppression due to chronic alcohol consumption. A low platelet count may be due to functional hypersplenism.
- **Clotting screen.** Prolonged INR and PT are indicative of impaired synthetic liver function, and occur in more advanced liver disease.
- **LFTs.** Liver function may be deranged or normal. In instances of apparently normal liver function, this may be the result of a profoundly cirrhotic liver that is no longer able to release liver enzymes due to a lack of remaining functional liver. Hypoalbuminaemia is a reflection of poor synthetic liver function.

TABLE 15.1 Patterns of abnormal liver function

	ALT	AST	GGT	ALP	CAUSES
Obstructive picture or cholestasis	↑	↑	↑↑	↑↑	Intrahepatic (e.g. PBC) Extrahepatic (e.g. gallstones, neoplasm of head of pancreas)
Hepatic picture	↑↑	↑↑	↑	↑	Alcohol Non-alcoholic fatty liver disease Drugs Acute/chronic viral hepatitis Ischaemic injury

- **U&Es.** Hyponatraemia is common in alcoholics. Also look for evidence of hepatorenal syndrome (deranged renal function).
- **Paracetamol and salicylate levels.** These should always be sent in cases of acute liver disease.
- **Viral serology** (e.g. hepatitis B and C, CMV, EBV and possibly HIV).
- **Immunoglobulins.** IgA, IgM and IgG may be raised in alcoholic liver disease and autoimmune disease.
- **Autoantibody screen.** This should include anti-mitochondrial antibody (AMA), anti-smooth muscle antibody (ASMA) and anti-nuclear antibody (ANA). The AMA level is elevated in more than 95% of patients with primary biliary cirrhosis (PBC).
- **USS and Dopplers of hepatic vessels.** Look for evidence of hepatomegaly (acutely) or a small shrunken cirrhotic liver (chronic), splenomegaly (portal hypertension), focal liver lesions (granulomas,

metastases, regenerative nodules, hepatocellular carcinoma) hepatic vein thrombosis and ascites.

- **Ascitic tap.** Send for an urgent Gram stain, cell count, MC&S and albumin. A WCC of > $250/mm^3$ indicates spontaneous bacterial peritonitis. If this is detected, discuss it with the microbiologist urgently and commence antibiotics.
- **Serum-ascites albumin gradient (SAAG).** This is used to help to determine the cause of ascites. Serum and ascitic albumin levels should be measured at the same time (*see* Box 15.2).

BOX 15.2 The serum ascites albumin gradient (SAAG)

SAAG = (albumin concentration of serum) − (albumin concentration of ascitic fluid)
A high gradient (> 1.1 g/dl) indicates that the ascites is due to portal hypertension.
Causes of a high SAAG include the following:
- high protein (> 2.5): heart failure
- low protein (< 2.5): cirrhosis of the liver, Budd–Chiari syndrome.

A low gradient (< 1.1 g/dl) indicates that the ascites is not associated with increased portal pressure.
Causes of a low SAAG include the following:
- nephrotic syndrome
- tuberculosis
- malignancy.

Further investigations
Iron studies
- **Ferritin, iron, TIBC and transferrin.** In iron overload states (e.g. haemochromatosis) the iron level will be raised and the TIBC will be low or normal, with an increased transferrin saturation. In other forms of liver disease the transferrin saturation is more likely to be decreased.

Caeruloplasmin
This is a copper-containing protein that normally binds 90% of the copper present in plasma. It is reduced in Wilson's disease, an autosomal recessive disorder in which copper accumulates in tissues which include the liver and brain.

Alpha fetoprotein

This is a marker of hepatocellular carcinoma or hepatic metastases. It may also be raised in other malignancies.

Alpha-1-antitrypsin

Deficiency of alpha-1-antitrypsin results in the breakdown of elastin in the liver and lungs by the enzyme elastase, leading to cirrhosis and chronic obstructive pulmonary disease.

Liver biopsy

This can be performed cutaneously or via the transjugular approach. Deranged clotting must be corrected before a cutaneous biopsy, with the INR < 1.3 and platelet count > 50 × 10⁹/l before the procedure is performed.

Diagnostic criteria in chronic liver disease

The Model for End-Stage Liver Disease (MELD) score

This is a scoring system for assessing the severity of chronic liver disease. It is useful for predicting mortality, determining the prognosis and prioritising the patient for liver transplantation. The score uses the patient's serum bilirubin and serum creatinine levels and their INR. It is calculated using the following formula:

$$\text{MELD} = 3.78 \, [\text{serum bilirubin (mg/dl)}] + 11.2 \, [\text{INR}] + 9.57 \, \text{serum creatinine (mg/dl)}] + 6.43.$$

The MELD score in hospitalised patients can predict their 3-month mortality as follows:
- ≥ 40: 71.3% mortality
- 30–39: 52.6% mortality
- 20–29: 19.6% mortality
- 10–19: 6.0% mortality
- ≤ 9: 1.9% mortality.

The Child's score

The Child's score has been developed primarily for use in cirrhotic patients who develop variceal bleeding or who are to undergo surgery. It is a useful tool for assessing mortality in this subset of patients.

TABLE 15.2 Child's grading of liver disease

GRADE	SERUM BILIRUBIN CONCENTRATION	SERUM ALBUMIN CONCENTRATION	ASCITES OR ENCEPHALOPATHY	OPERATIVE MORTALITY
A	Normal	> 35g/l	None	2%
B	20–50 µmol/l	30–35 g/l	Mild	10%
C	> 50 µmol/l	< 30 g/l	Severe, uncontrolled	50%

Management

General measures

1 **Complete abstinence from alcohol.** If cirrhosis has been caused by alcohol, the mortality is dramatically increased from 30% to about 70%.
2 **Nutrition.** All patients should be assessed by a dietician.
3 **Drugs.** Avoid the use of NSAIDS, sedatives and opiates.

Specific treatment for decompensation

Ascites
1 Fluid restriction to < 1.5 l/day; caution is needed with regard to intravascular depletion and renal impairment.
2 Review by a dietician.
3 Daily weights and measurement of abdominal girth.
4 Diuretics: Spironolactone 100 mg by mouth once a day, gradually increasing the dose to a maximum of 400 mg by mouth once a day. Furosemide 40 mg by mouth once a day can be added in if there is little response. Up-titrate to a maximum dose of 120 mg by mouth once a day.
5 Diagnostic ascitic tap (see below).
6 Therapeutic paracentesis with concomitant intravenous human albumin solution may be tried if there is rapidly accumulating or tense ascites. Check the bloods for clotting and platelet results first. It is usually safe to drain ascites if the INR is < 1.3 and the platelet count is > 50×10^9/l (*see* Chapter 3).
7 Monitor the patient carefully for signs of intravascular depletion following paracentesis.
   GI bleeding secondary to varices (*see* Chapter 5).

Encephalopathy
- Exclude non-hepatic causes of altered mental function.
- A serum ammonia level may be useful, so the lab should be contacted to arrange this.
- Correct precipitants.
- Lactulose – this inhibits the formation of colonic bacteria, and thereby

inhibits ammonia production. The initial dose is 30 ml by mouth daily to lead to two to four loose stools per day.

- Antibiotics (e.g. neomycin, metronidazole and oral vancomycin) may reduce the colonic bacterial load. These are usually used as second-line agents.
- Patients with severe encephalopathy (i.e. grade 3 or 4) who are at risk for aspiration should undergo prophylactic endotracheal intubation. They are best managed in the intensive care unit.

Spontaneous bacterial peritonitis
1 Diagnostic tap.
2 Antibiotics if the WCC is > 250 cells/mm^3. Discuss this with the microbiologist. One regimen is cefuroxime 1.5 g/8 hours + metronidazole 500 mg once a day until sensitivities are known.

Important tips
Alcohol liaison service
All patients with alcoholic liver disease must be advised to stop drinking alcohol. They should also be referred to an alcohol liaison team for regular follow-up and advice.

Previous records
Patients with known cirrhotic liver disease are likely to have had previous investigations. Old notes are extremely important, as they will provide you with information about previous OGDs which may give an indication as to whether varices are present. In addition, note whether the patient has had previous USS and alpha fetoprotein measurements.

Information to have to hand for ward rounds
1 Up-to-date bloods, including FBC, U&Es, LFTs, clotting and alpha fetoprotein.
2 The results of the infection screen, with any up-to-date microbiology.
3 The results of ascitic fluid aspiration.
4 The results of the most recent USS (and OGD and/or MRI if undertaken), or the date when this investigation is booked.
5 A comprehensive medical history, including alcohol use, drug use, tattoos, etc.
6 Observation chart for temperature and haemodynamic status, GCS score, grade of encephalopathy, weight and stool and urine chart.

16

Acute pancreatitis

Epidemiology

Acute pancreatitis is particularly common in Western populations, with alcoholic pancreatitis being more prevalent in the USA, and gallstone-related pancreatitis occurring more frequently in Europe. The incidence of acute pancreatitis in the UK is rising, with a current hospital admission rate of 9.8 per year per 100 000 members of the population.

Aetiology

Gallstones and alcohol are the major causes of acute pancreatitis. The mnemonic GET SMASHED is widely cited as an aide-memoire for the various causes of the disease:

- **Gallstones**
- **Ethanol**
- **Trauma**
- **Steroids**
- **Mumps**
- **Autoimmune**
- **Scorpion venom**
- **Hypercalcaemia/hypertriglyceridaemia/ hypothermia**
- **ERCP**
- **Drugs** (e.g. azathioprine and sulphonamides).

The inflammatory process that is seen in acute pancreatitis is allied to several cytokines, including TNF, IL-1, IL-6 and IL-8. Studies have also shown that activation of the enzyme trypsin is an initial step in the development of the disease.

Clinical presentation

Patients typically present with abdominal pain, which is commonly dull in character, and often extremely severe. It is central in nature and radiates through to the back. The patient may feel nauseated, or vomit or complain of diarrhoea. Examination findings may demonstrate the presence of a fever and tachycardia. A blue discoloration of the umbilicus (Cullen's sign) or a brown-red discoloration of the flanks (Grey Turner's sign) may be noted. The latter is due to the spread of retroperitoneal blood.

Initial investigations

- **FBC.** A raised WCC may be present, and can be used in the risk stratification in accordance with Ranson's and Glasgow criteria. The platelet count may be high or low. Normocytic anaemia may indicate an alcohol-related aetiology causing bone-marrow suppression.
- **U&Es.** A raised urea concentration (> 16 mmol/l) forms part of the risk stratification of the Glasgow and Ranson's criteria.
- **LFTs.** Deranged liver function may indicate an underlying aetiology of gallstone pancreatitis. ALT may be elevated to two to three times the upper normal limit. Both ALT and AST form part of the Glasgow and Ranson's criteria. Hypoalbuminaemia is also a marker of disease severity.
- **Amylase.** Activity of this enzyme is often elevated in acute pancreatitis. However, it may be normal, and furthermore it is not specific.
- **Bone profile.** Hypocalcaemia (serum calcium concentration of < 2 mmol/l) is a marker of disease severity.
- **CRP.** This is often elevated, but is not specific for the condition.
- **Serum lipase.** Measurement often demonstrates a rise in serum lipase levels within 4–8 hours after the onset of acute pancreatitis.
- **Glucose.** Raised glucose levels may indicate pancreatic dysfunction.
- **Clotting screen.** Clotting dysfunction may represent poor synthetic liver function, and is especially important in individuals with a heavy alcohol intake. DIC may also occur in the context of extremely severe acute pancreatitis. If DIC is suspected, a serum fibrinogen level should be sent.
- **ABG.** Hypoxia to a level of < 8 kPa is a marker of disease severity.
- **ECG.** It is important to exclude atypical presentations of myocardial ischaemia.
- **CXR.** Elevated hemidiaphragms, small pleural effusions and basal atelectasis may occur in patients with acute pancreatitis.
- **AXR.** More commonly the abdominal film may be completely normal.

A localised ileus may be present. Features of chronic pancreatic changes may be present in the form of calcifications in the pancreas.

The severity of acute pancreatitis is demonstrated by the following Ranson criteria markers:

- white cell count > 15×10^9/l
- urea concentration > 16 mmol/l
- calcium concentration < 2 mmol/l
- albumin concentration < 32 g/l
- glucose concentration > 10 mmol/l
- PO_2 < 8 kPa
- AST > 200 IU/l
- LDH > 600 IU/l
- CRP > 150 mg/l.

Severity assessment is also based on the APACHE II criteria, with a score of > 8 indicating an 11–18% risk of mortality.

Measurement of CRP with a peak of > 210 mg/l on day 2–4, or > 120 mg/l at the end of the first week is another useful marker of disease severity in patients with acute pancreatitis.

Further investigations

USS

An ultrasound scan is a cheap and non-invasive initial imaging investigation. Although it is not highly sensitive, its specificity is high. As well as identifying the presence of acute pancreatitis, it may also diagnose an underlying aetiology.

CT scan

Abdominal CT scanning is always indicated in individuals with suspected acute pancreatitis. The CT may reveal pancreatic enlargement, irregular contours and streaking of peripancreatic fat tissue. Intraperitoneal or retroperitoneal free fluid may also be present. This fluid may be haemorrhagic in the context of necrotising pancreatitis. However, the CT may be completely normal in acute pancreatitis.

An additional severity screen is based on the CT Severity Index, which utilises a combined score derived from the CT appearance (Balthazar score) and necrosis percentage (*see* Tables 16.1 and 16.2).

TABLE 16.1 Balthazar CT grading of acute pancreatitis

BALTHAZAR GRADE	APPEARANCE ON CT	NUMBER OF CT GRADE POINTS
A	Normal CT	0
B	Focal or diffuse enlargement of the pancreas	1
C	Pancreatic gland abnormalities and peripancreatic inflammation	2
D	Fluid collection in a single location	3
E	Two or more fluid collections and/ or gas bubbles in or adjacent to the pancreas	4

TABLE 16.2 Grading of severity of acute pancreatitis according to necrosis percentage

NECROSIS PERCENTAGE	NUMBER OF POINTS
No necrosis	0
0–30% necrosis	2
30–50% necrosis	4
> 50% necrosis	6

MRI

MRI can detect the same findings as CT imaging, but with the additional benefit of good-quality biliary imaging for obstruction. MRI is also useful in patients with poor renal function that precludes the use of contrast in CT imaging.

Angiography

Pancreatic enzymes can cause the erosion of blood vessels in the proximity of the pancreas. This can result in life-threatening haemorrhage. Angiography can be used in conjunction with interventional techniques for selective embolisation of blood vessels. Selective embolisation is only available in centres that have interventional radiology services.

Management

Acute pancreatitis is usually managed by surgeons. However, it is important to be able to recognise the presentation and initial management steps, as in severe cases this condition can rapidly become fatal.

Medical management

Initial management relies on aggressive resuscitation measures, particularly in the setting of sepsis and shocked patients. The patient should also be made nil by mouth, and have a nasogastric tube inserted.

- **Fluids.** Patients often become severely intravascularly depleted due to third-space losses. Fluid replacement should be intravenous. A nasogastric tube should also be placed on free drainage. These patients are often extremely unwell, and it may be advisable to insert a central venous catheter, which will also guide fluid resuscitation. In addition, a urinary catheter should be placed to ensure accurate fluid balance assessment.
- **Nutrition.** Enteral nutrition has been shown to be highly beneficial in the management of acute pancreatitis. This is primarily due to the patient's limited oral intake and the existence of a catabolic state. It allows for significant pancreatic rest and helps to prevent the absorption of endotoxins and cytokines from the GI tract.
- **Antibiotics.** The use of antibiotics remains controversial. In cases of necrotising pancreatitis, antibiotic therapy has been shown to be useful. Buchler *et al.*[1] demonstrated that the use of imipenem, ofloxacin and ciprofloxacin provided sufficient tissue penetration and bactericidal action. It is advisable to consult local trust antibiotic guidelines as well as to discuss such cases with a microbiologist.
- **ERCP.** This procedure has been utilised in the management of acute pancreatitis secondary to gallstones, and in the case of pseudocyst formation. Contraindications to the use of ERCP-based drainage include the presence of varices, impaired coagulation and significant thickening of the cyst wall.

Surgical management

Surgical management is now rarely used in cases of acute pancreatitis, as the surgical role has diminished with the advent of minimally invasive interventional techniques. However, surgical necrosectomy is still performed. In cases where pseudocyst formation is extensive, surgery may also prove beneficial.

Daily monitoring/investigations

1   Close observation of vital signs.
2   Blood cultures whenever there is a temperature spike > 38 °C.
3   Daily examination, looking specifically for signs of necrotising pancreatitis,

abdominal tenderness and signs of sepsis. Make an assessment of fluid balance.

4   FBC, U&Es, CRP, LFTs and clotting on alternate days.

Important tips

Microbiology

Antibiotic treatment may be appropriate. It is of particular importance to consider antibiotic cover in patients who are undergoing ERCP. We recommend that you either discuss this with your microbiologists or consult your local guidelines.

Cannulas

Intravenous cannulas are a common source of infection in hospitals. Ensure that you change the cannula every 3 days, and inspect cannula sites daily for early signs of local infection. Write the date of insertion on the cannula dressing, and record this in the notes to avoid confusion.

Scoring systems

It is worth using the scoring systems described in this chapter. They will help to identify the patients who are likely to require the most support, as well as identifying the appropriate management settings for patients (i.e. HDU or ITU).

Dieticians

Discussion of cases of patients with severe acute pancreatitis is important, as this will ensure that these patients are commenced on the correct enteral nutrition programmes. Close liaison with the dietician will help to provide better care for the patient.

Surgeons

Acute pancreatitis is usually managed by the surgeons. In some trusts the care is shared between the surgeons and physicians. It is important to discuss patient cases with the surgeons early on in the admission.

Future advice

Any patient with acute pancreatitis that has been caused by alcohol excess must be warned about the dangers of continuing to consume alcohol. It is worth discussing with the patient whether they would like to be put in contact with either the alcohol liaison team or the drugs and alcohol addiction unit.

Information to have to hand for ward rounds

1 Up-to-date bloods, including FBC, U&Es, LFTs, CRP and clotting.
2 The results of the USS and/or CT abdomen.
3 Up-to-date microbiology results.
4 The current antibiotic regimen and length of course to date, if applicable.
5 Observation chart for temperature and haemodynamic status.

Reference

1 Buchler M, Malfertheiner P, Friess H *et al.* Human pancreatic tissue concentration of bactericidal antibiotics. *Gastroenterology* 1992; **103:** 1902–8.

Further reading

• Leser HG, Gross V, Scheibenbogen C *et al.* Elevation of serum interleukin-6 concentration precedes acute-phase response and reflects severity in acute pancreatitis. *Gastroenterology* 1991; **101:** 782–5.
• Banks P and Freeman M. Practice guidelines in acute pancreatitis. *American Journal of Gastroenterology* 2006; **101:** 2379–400.
• Balthazar EJ, Robinson DL, Megibow AJ *et al.* Acute pancreatitis: value of CT in establishing prognosis. *Radiology* 1990; **174:** 331–6.
• Wilson C, Heads A, Shenkin A *et al.* C-reactive protein, antiproteases and complement factors as objective markers of severity in acute pancreatitis. *British Journal of Surgery* 1989; **76:** 177–81.
• Buchler M, Malfertheiner P, Friess H *et al.* Human pancreatic tissue concentration of bactericidal antibiotics. *Gastroenterology* 1992; **103:** 1902–8.

17

Chronic pancreatitis

Epidemiology

Chronic pancreatitis is particularly common in the Western world. Males are more frequently affected than females, although hypertriglyceridaemia-associated pancreatitis is more common in women.

The annual incidence in the UK is 1 per 100 000 members of the population, with a prevalence of 3 per 100 000. The average age of onset is around 40 years.

Aetiology

Chronic pancreatitis arises as a result of prolonged damage to the structure and function of the pancreas itself, and is often seen following continued inflammatory insult. In Europe the predominant cause is significant alcohol misuse. Additional causes include autoimmune damage (SLE, autoimmune pancreatitis, primary biliary cirrhosis, Sjogren's syndrome), hyperparathyroidism and hypertriglyceridaemia. In some instances the cause may not be known.

From a genetic perspective, the cystic fibrosis transmembrane regulator (CFTR) gene is implicated in disease pathogenesis, with the delta F508 mutation causing impaired cAMP regulation of chloride channels, thickened secretions and subsequent pancreatic duct blockage. Additional genes of interest include SPINK1.

Clinical presentation

Patients present with mid- to upper abdominal pain which usually bears no relationship to eating. There is commonly a prolonged history of multiple similar episodes of abdominal pain. These episodes of abdominal pain may last for several hours, with patients obtaining some improvement in their pain by leaning forward. Malabsorption results in diarrhoea/steatorrhoea, weight loss and anorexia. Patients may also present with features of diabetes due to pancreatic dysfunction.

Initial investigations

- **FBC.** This is commonly normal. However, it may reveal a normocytic anaemia of chronic disease. A low platelet count may be present in the setting of chronic alcohol misuse.
- **U&Es.** This is likely to be normal. However, it may show evidence of biochemical dehydration with raised creatinine and urea levels.
- **LFTs.** Alcohol excess may result in abnormalities of liver function. However, in the late stages of liver disease one often sees 'normalisation' of liver function values, due to cirrhosis. Hypoalbuminaemia may result from malnutrition.
- **Serum calcium levels.** These are usually normal in the setting of chronic pancreatitis, in contrast to the situation in acute pancreatitis.
- **Amylase.** Activity of this enzyme is usually normal, or may be slightly elevated. Amylase has no diagnostic value in chronic pancreatitis.
- **CRP.** Infection should be ruled out, especially in the context of deranged liver function.
- **Autoimmune screen.** ESR, ANA, anti-SMA, rheumatoid factor and IgG4 may be elevated in cases of autoimmune chronic pancreatitis.
- **Fasting serum glucose levels.** Chronic pancreatitis may result in impairment of pancreatic function and subsequent diabetes. Patients may also require oral glucose tolerance testing.
- **CXR.** In the setting of acute abdominal pain, patients should undergo an erect CXR to help to exclude gastrointestinal perforation.
- **AXR.** Around 30% of patients with chronic pancreatitis show evidence of calcification of the pancreas on a plain abdominal film.
- **Faecal fat.** Excretion of more than 7 g of fat in stool per day is abnormal and indicates malabsorption.
- **Faecal elastase.** Normal exocrine pancreatic function should produce a level of > 200 µg/g. Levels below this value suggest that there is reduced exocrine pancreatic function.

Further investigations

USS

An abdominal USS is a cheap and non-invasive investigation that is readily available. In addition to looking at other causes of abdominal pain, it allows imaging of the pancreas to look for pancreatic calcification, pancreatic and peripancreatic oedema, and pseudocysts.

CT

An abdominal CT allows the detection of enlargement, atrophy, calcification and pseudocyst formation with a higher sensitivity and specificity than can be achieved with ultrasound.

MRCP

MRCP is the gold standard of imaging techniques, with the highest sensitivity and specificity. It allows accurate anatomical imaging of the pancreas and biliary tree to aid diagnosis.

ERCP

As well as being an accurate imaging modality, ERCP has the additional benefit of being able to take histological samples and brushings of the ducts for cytological investigation. Unfortunately, this procedure also carries many risks of iatrogenic complication, including pancreatitis.

EUS

EUS has a similar sensitivity to that of ERCP, but with reduced rates of iatrogenic complications.

Management

The treatment of chronic pancreatitis, like that of acute pancreatitis, often relies on focusing on the underlying cause.

Medical management

- **General management.** Precipitating factors should be removed, especially if the aetiology is alcohol. Patients should also be advised to stop smoking, and should avoid eating large meals, and especially meals with a high fat content.
- **Analgesia.** Pain is particularly problematic for these patients. They often require high doses of analgesia, and are often trialled on amitriptyline and gabapentin. In some extreme cases of uncontrolled pain, studies have demonstrated the potential for use of coeliac plexus neurolysis to destroy the afferent nerve supply.

- **Nutrition.** Due to the malabsorption associated with this disease, patients often become malnourished. It is therefore advisable to discuss such patients with a dietician in order to obtain advice on dietary supplementation.
- **Pancreatic enzyme supplementation.** Enzyme supplementation, as well as enhancing nutritional status, has the added benefit of improving pain control.
- **Steatorrhoea.** Avoidance of foods with a high fat content is advisable. Patients can also be given lipase, and may require supplementation of the fat-soluble vitamins (A, D, E and K).

Surgical management

As in the case of acute pancreatitis, surgery is employed in cases where pseudocysts are complicating the disease.

The presence of strictures or stones within the pancreatic ductal system may be amenable to endoscopic intervention. However, surgical intervention is reserved for those cases where these techniques have failed.

Daily monitoring and investigations

Patients with chronic pancreatitis are at risk of developing diabetes as well as biliary tract and duodenal obstruction, and should therefore be monitored for such complications accordingly.

Important tips

Cannulas

Intravenous cannulas are a common source of infection in hospitals. Ensure that you change the cannula every 3 days, and inspect cannula sites daily for early signs of local infection. Write the date of insertion on the cannula dressing, and record this in the notes to avoid confusion.

Previous records

Review the patient's case notes, particularly for details of previous admissions and investigations. This will aid the planning of further investigations if these are required, as well as allowing appropriate management of the patient.

Future advice

All patients must be advised to abstain completely from alcohol, irrespective of the aetiology of the disease. They should also be advised to reduce the size of their meals and avoid foods with a high fat content.

Dietician
Patients will benefit from advice and follow-up from a dietician to ensure that they are receiving their nutritional requirements. They should be assessed as inpatients, and followed up in the community if there are any further issues.

Changes in clinical picture
In patients with a known history of chronic pancreatitis, a change in the pattern or severity of pain may denote pancreatic cancer, and must be investigated.

Surgical advice
Chronic pancreatitis is usually managed by the physicians (whereas acute pancreatitis is usually surgically managed). Patients should be discussed with the surgeons so that they are aware of the patient in the event of deterioration during the admission.

Information to have to hand for ward rounds
1 Up-to-date bloods, including FBC, U&Es, LFTs, CRP and ESR.
2 Faecal elastase results.
3 The results of the most recent imaging (USS, CT, AXR, CXR, etc.).
4 Pain score.
5 Observation chart for temperature and haemodynamic status.
6 Stool chart.

Further reading
- Noone PG, Zhou Z, Silverman LM *et al*. Cystic fibrosis gene mutations and pancreatitis risk: relation to epithelial ion transport and trypsin inhibitor gene mutations. *Gastroenterology* 2001; **121**: 1310–19.

18

Pancreatic cancer

Epidemiology

Pancreatic cancer has been shown to commonly occur in black populations in the USA, in Koreans, and in the Maori population of New Zealand. The median age of diagnosis is 69 years in Caucasian populations and 65 years in black populations.

Aetiology

Numerous risk factors are associated with the development of pancreatic cancer. The condition is more common in males and in older individuals. It can occur in association with chronic pancreatitis, diabetes mellitus, Peutz–Jeghers syndrome and HNPCC. Lifestyle risk factors include smoking, chronic alcohol misuse and a low dietary intake of fruit and vegetables. From a genetic perspective, K-ras oncogenic mutations have been associated with the condition, and the p16 and TP53 tumour suppressor genes are also commonly inactivated in pancreatic cancer.

Clinical presentation

Symptomatology is dependent largely on the location of the tumour, with tumours of the head and body of the pancreas, for example, resulting in compression of the bile duct, coeliac nerves and duodenum. Tumours of the head of the pancreas often result in painless jaundice. In general, pancreatic cancer is associated with abdominal pain, back pain, weight loss allied to malabsorption, and diabetes mellitus. Tumours of the pancreatic tail are associated with pain in the left or left upper side of the abdomen.

Initial investigations

- **FBC.** Patients may show evidence of a normochromic, normocytic anaemia. The platelet count may be elevated.
- **U&Es.** Baseline renal function is useful, as patients are likely to require CT imaging and the use of contrast.
- **LFTs.** Evidence of obstructive jaundice may be noted with raised serum bilirubin levels and elevated alkaline phosphatase activity. The transaminases are less likely to be elevated.
- **Albumin.** Advanced-stage disease may be associated with significantly malnourished patients, resulting in hypoalbuminaemia.
- **CA 19-9.** This is elevated in up to 85% of cases of pancreatic cancer. Unfortunately, CA 19-9 is least sensitive for small early-stage pancreatic carcinomas. Pre-operative CA 19-9 is often used as a prognostic marker, with particularly high levels indicating a poorer outcome.
- **AXR.** Occasionally, chronic pancreatitis may result in calcifications in the pancreas which may be observed on X-ray.
- **CXR.** Ideally this should be an erect CXR, which will also help to exclude other causes of abdominal pain, such as perforation. In addition, look closely for evidence of pulmonary metastases which, if found, warrant staging CT.

Further investigations

CT abdomen

The gold standard diagnostic investigation is an abdominal CT scan. Discuss the case with a radiologist to ensure that the correct type of CT is undertaken. A triple-phase spiral CT has an accuracy of approximately 90%. Imaging will also aid the surgeon if there is any chance of resection. Tissue biopsies allow a histological diagnosis to be made, and can be obtained via CT guidance or endoscopic ultrasound. An abdominal CT scan will also help to demonstrate evidence of metastases, which commonly occur to the liver.

ERCP

This procedure has the advantage of use as a diagnostic tool (through imaging combined with biopsy and brushings), combined with therapeutic modalities. If there is evidence of obstructive jaundice, an ERCP with subsequent stent placement is desirable. Unfortunately, these benefits do not come without risks, and stent placement is associated with a 5–10% risk of complications, some of which are serious.

MRCP
This is a useful non-invasive imaging modality for the diagnosis of small lesions that are not picked up on CT. It can produce high-quality images of the pancreatic duct and biliary tree.

EUS
Endoscopic ultrasound is the most sensitive and specific diagnostic tool for pancreatic cancer. Unfortunately, it is usually only available in specialist centres. EUS can be used as an imaging tool to assess whether a tumour is resectable, as an aid to staging, and also for taking biopsies.

Management
Medical management
- **Analgesia.** This is an important area of management, especially in palliative patients, for whom pain can be a significant problem. It is often worth discussing issues of analgesia with either the pain control team or the palliative care team.
- **Nausea and vomiting.** Patients may be nauseated due to the underlying disease process, or due to opiate analgesics or as a result of chemotherapeutic agents. In cases where simple anti-emetics fail to control the symptoms, expert advice should be sought from the palliative care team.
- **Jaundice.** This is often treated with stent insertion at ERCP to relieve the obstruction caused by the tumour. This is especially important in palliative cases where patients are suffering with cholangitis or pruritus.
- **Chemotherapy.** Non-resectable cancers refer to those cases where the tumour is associated with involvement of the superior mesenteric arterial/venous supply or coeliac axis. The treatment of choice in such situations is chemoradiation with fluorouracil-based therapy, which was demonstrated to be significantly efficacious by the Gastrointestinal Tumour Study Group in the 1980s.[1]

Surgical management
The management of pancreatic cancer is dependent on the extent of tumour spread. Cancers that are deemed to be resectable include those which do not involve the superior mesenteric arterial/venous supply or coeliac axis. Studies have also demonstrated that adjuvant chemoradiation-based therapy is beneficial in resectable cases.

Novel therapies
The pathogenesis and subsequent spread of pancreatic cancer depends

upon several growth factors, inflammatory mediators and genetically based mutations. Therapies targeted at these molecular levels may therefore show promise in the treatment of the condition. Such agents include epidermal growth factor receptor antagonists (e.g. ZD1839 and OSI-774) as well as vascular growth factor inhibitors (e.g. bevacizumab).

Daily monitoring/investigations

1 Close observation of vital signs.
2 Blood cultures whenever there is a temperature spike of > 38 °C, as there may be underlying biliary sepsis.
3 Daily examination.
4 Twice weekly bloods, including FBC, LFTs and CRP.

Important tips

Palliative care

Discuss all patients who have a confirmed diagnosis with the palliative care team early on. The prognosis for pancreatic cancer is extremely poor, and good-quality management is essential for patients and their families. In cases where curative resection is to be undertaken, the palliative care team may also have a useful role in pain control and the management of nausea and vomiting.

ERCP and stent insertion

If the patient is to have a stent inserted at ERCP, ensure that they have had a recent clotting screen and correct any abnormalities of clotting function. Prophylactic antibiotics should also be prescribed before ERCP, and in addition prior to stent insertion. Check the local hospital guidelines on which antibiotics to use.

Information to have to hand for ward rounds

1 Up-to-date bloods, including FBC, U&Es, LFTs and CRP.
2 Tumour markers.
3 The results of the most recent imaging, or the date when it is booked.
4 Observation chart for temperature and haemodynamic status.

Reference

1 Moertel CG, Frytak S, Hahn RG *et al*. Therapy of locally unresectable pancreatic carcinoma: a randomized comparison of high dose

(6000 rads) radiation alone, moderate dose radiation (4000 rads + 5-fluorouracil), and high dose radiation + 5-fluorouracil. *Cancer* 1981; **48:** 1705–10.

Further reading

- Papageorgio C and Perry MC. Epidermal growth factor receptor-targeted therapy for pancreatic cancer. *Cancer Investigation* 2007; **25:** 647–57.
- Kindler HL, Friberg G, Singh DA *et al.* Phase II trial of bevacizumab plus gemcitabine in patients with advanced pancreatic cancer. *Journal of Clinical Oncology* 2005; **23:** 8033–40.

Index